Finding Out About
VICTORIAN PUBLIC HEALTH AND HOUSING

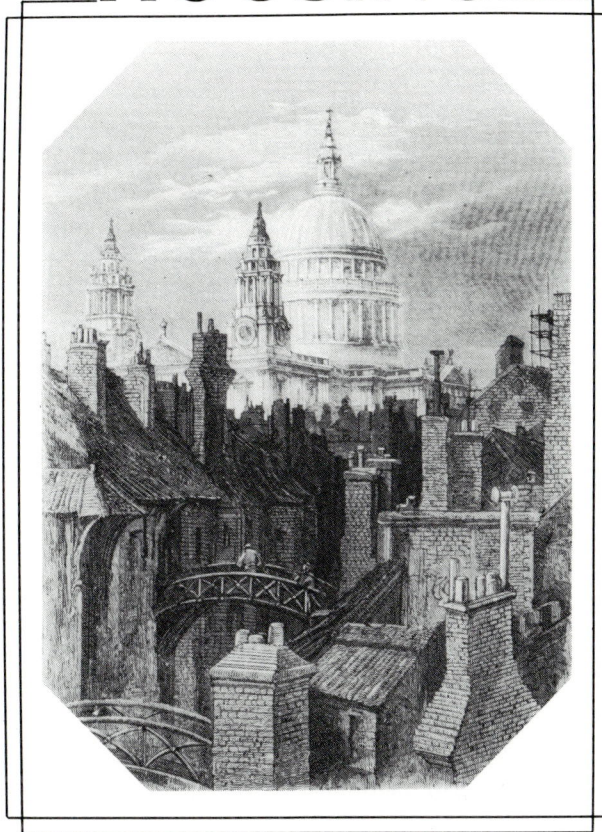

Michael Rawcliffe

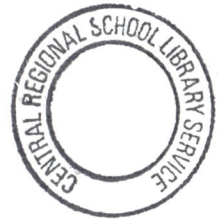

B.T. Batsford Limited, London

Contents

© Michael Rawcliffe 1987
First published 1987

Typeset by Tek-Art Ltd, Kent
and printed in Great Britain by
R J Acford Ltd,
Chichester, Sussex
for the publishers
B.T. Batsford Limited,
4 Fitzhardinge Street
London W1H 0AH

ISBN 0 7134 5050 9

ACKNOWLEDGMENTS

The Author and Publishers would like to thank the following for their kind permission to reproduce illustrations: The British Museum (National Photographic Record) and London Borough of Tower Hamlets for page 24; Croydon Public Libraries for pages 10, 28 and 41; Oxford Central Library for pages 23, 29 and 33 (top); *Punch* for page 16; Sheffield City Library for pages 8, 28 and 41. Illustrations on pages 3, 5, 17, 20, and 30 are from the author's collection. The diagram on page 37 and the map on page 44 were drawn by R.F. Brien.

Cover Illustrations

The colour engraving is of Manchester in the 1840s; the black and white photograph shows London slums backing on the south bank of the Thames, c. 1860, while the notice shows that by the later part of the century it was possible in some areas to be connected to the main sewers.

TS

This book is ~~~~~~~~~~~ on or before

Introduction

A person living in modern Britain takes many things for granted. When we want a wash a regular supply of water is available through the tap, and we do not need to worry about whether the water is unsafe or polluted. Equally, when we flush the toilet a ready supply of water clears the pan into the main drains. Occasionally things go wrong, but this is usually due to an internal fault such as a valve, washer or burst pipe, rather than a fault in the system.

Similarly, the vast majority of houses and flats today have either gas or electricity which provides for cooking, lighting, and possibly heating. When we go outside, the streets are lit, the roads and pavements are looked after and the dustbins regularly emptied.

When we sit down to a meal the bread, the milk and other foodstuffs are safe and can be trusted not to harm us. In fact, we probably don't think twice about it, and are only concerned if the bread is stale or the milk is warm.

However, this has not always been so. At the beginning of the nineteenth century few homes had an internal supply of water or an internal toilet, and a continuous supply of water was not general before 1900. Similarly, houses or rooms which the poor could afford to rent were always in short supply and overcrowding was common in the towns. Even new buildings did not have to be built to minimum standards or provide basic facilities.

Mooreland Road, Bromley, Kent. In 1868 the houses were served only by pumps or well-water and had no internal sanitation.

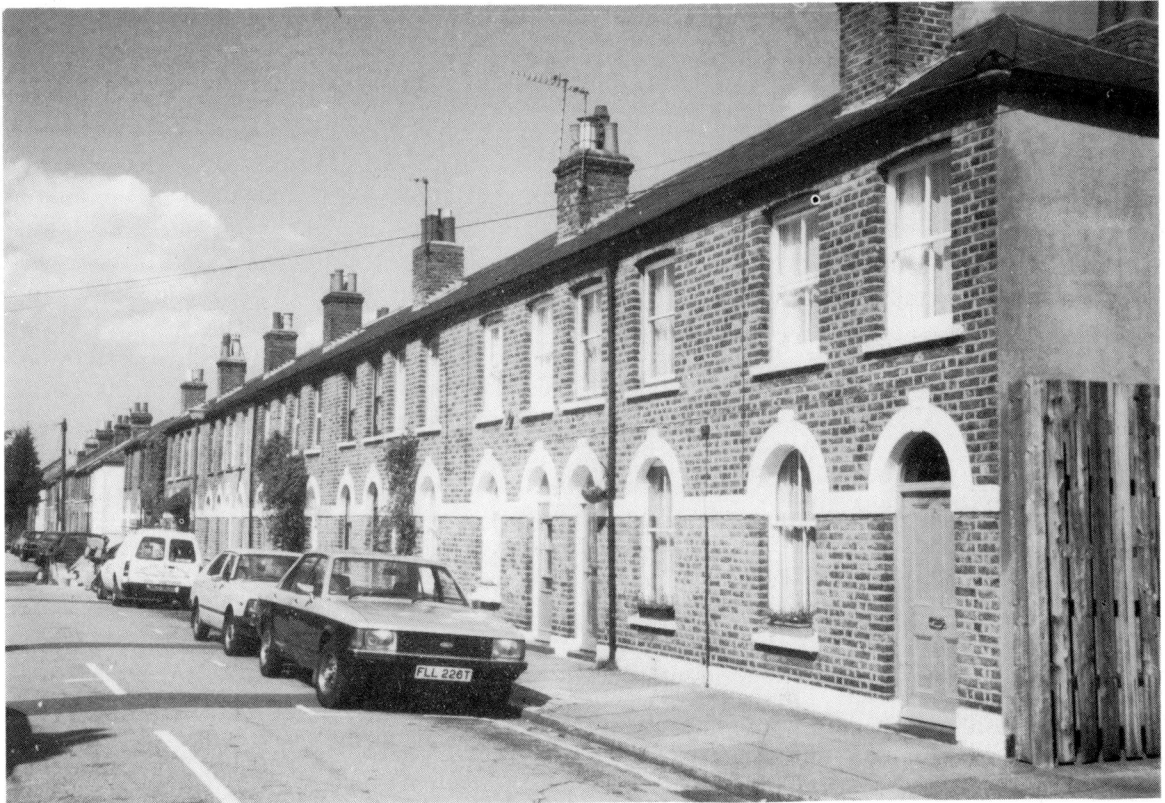

Many people felt that this was right and that one should be able to choose rather than being told, or required by law, to do certain things. Reforms and improvements were often expensive and were frequently opposed by people living in less densely populated areas, who would have to bear the higher charges.

The largest problems were to be found in London which in the first half of the nineteenth century annually absorbed numbers equal to that of a large town. As the population rapidly grew the towns and cities could not cope. There was no central town authority to take control and, as we shall see, the problems of inadequate housing, overcrowding, disease and pollution of the air and water increased. However, it was often death which brought home the problems. "King Cholera", which visited Britain on several occasions, was no respecter of persons and bred fear amongst all. Death produced the background against which the arguments of the reformers were heard, and acted upon.

By the end of the century many improvements had been made. The death rate had more than halved and there were now local authorities which could raise money through the rates and employ officials such as sanitary officers to enforce the laws which had been passed. In 1900 a lot had still to be done, but the foundations of public health had been laid.

This book is primarily about the problems faced by the large towns and, in particular, London. This is largely because by 1851 the majority of people lived in urban areas. The examples chosen may not be from your area, but they will provide the stimulus and give examples for you to find out what conditions were like in your area and how change came about.

This section is intended to give you suggestions for the type of sources that you will find in your area.

1. PEOPLE

Very few people living today were born in Victorian Britain, but parents and grandparents may well remember things which were told to them many years ago.

Your first contact will be your teacher, who will be able to give you details of your nearest local history library or record office. The librarians there will be helpful but they get many requests for help and are very busy. Thus it is essential that you have a clear idea of what you want to find out and a general idea of the type of materials which will be available. Always check the opening days and hours, and if you are travelling some distance it is best to write first giving as much information as you can. Take a notebook and pencil with you and some loose change in case you need to xerox any material that you want copied.

2. THE AREA TO BE STUDIED

If you live in a village the older houses may still remain, but in a town much redevelopment is likely to have taken place. Nevertheless, it is essential that you walk the area with a map (see 3b) in order to locate the main features. Many questions will be raised such as what stood on the site of the railway station or the Victorian Town Hall and where would older houses have been which once surrounded the medieval Parish Church? This will be useful when you read about the parts of the town which had the greatest public health problems.

3. VISUAL MATERIAL

a) Old photographs. The library is likely to have a good collection of Victorian photographs. You may find ones of streets and buildings which still exist. What changes have taken place? Very few photographs exist showing the interiors of ordinary houses, and many photographs of people will show people posing in their best clothes. It is always worth asking yourself why a particular photograph was taken.

b) Maps. By the middle of the nineteenth century

the Ordnance Survey had produced a wide range of maps of the country at the 1-inch, 6-inch and 25-inch scale. These were frequently updated and this will enable you to trace change over time.

c) Prints and paintings. Before the photograph, line drawings were frequently used in books and newspapers. *The Illustrated London News* and *Punch* contain many illustrations which will be useful. Edwin Chadwick's *Sanitary Conditions of the Labouring Population*, published in 1842, made an enormous impact, in part because it was illustrated.

4. WRITTEN SOURCES

The local library will indicate the most useful sources to you.

a) Local histories. These are always a good starting point and, even if the text is difficult, they may contain some useful maps, illustrations, extracts or ideas which you can follow up.

b) Local directories. These are a valuable and common source, as every county has its Victorian directory, and many towns have them, too. Kelly's *Post Office Directory* is the most common. They were regularly updated and provide detail on every town and village, giving the population, major residents, traders and professional people and other local detail.

c) Advertisements. They will enable you to chart changing attitudes towards public health. They often showed builders' advertisements stressing well-drained sites for their houses, plumbers illustrating the latest sinks and basins and gas-fitters advertising their trade.

d) Documents. These were written at the time for practical use. You will find in the library examples such as the Minutes of the Local Board of Health and the reports of the Medical Officer of Health.

e) Diaries and memoirs. These will not be written specifically on public health or housing but may contain references to epidemics, deaths, or lack of water.

c) Census material. The first national census was in 1801, and it has been carried out every ten years since then, except for 1941. It is particulary useful for giving examples of overcrowding and the occupations, ages and place of birth of those who

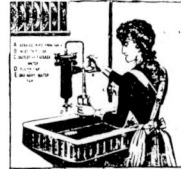

Berkefield Filters – a late nineteenth-century magazine advertisement. Why do the manufacturers list to whom they supply their product?

lived in particular houses. The latest census available is that of 1881, because of the hundred-year rule on the release of personal information. The census data is usually on microfilm in the local library.

5. OBJECTS

The local museum may have a useful collection of Victoriana and you may come across the village pump or a well on your investigations.

6. ROADS, FIELD AND INN NAMES

These may give us useful clues to the past. Hospital Road, Gas Works Road, etc. may indicate their location in the nineteenth century, whilst reformers such as Peel, Chadwick or Gladstone might be honoured by street names or public houses.

The Industrial Town

THE SPEED OF GROWTH

In 1801 London had a population of just under a million. No other city had a population of more than 100,000. By 1851 the figures were as follows:

London	2,250,000
Liverpool	375,155
Manchester	250,409
Birmingham	232,841
Leeds	172,270

What do all five cities have in common?

A.J. Langford wrote in *A Century of Birmingham Life*, published in 1870, that one

. . . could expect to find a street of houses in the Autumn where he saw his horse at grass in the Spring.

How rapidly did your town grow in the nineteenth century?

A VIEW OF MANCHESTER

Manchester was the first industrial town based upon factories, and before public transport developed the workers lived near their place of work. At first Manchester was unique, and there were those who felt that the dirt was a necessary cost if wealth was to be made. Its population increased sixfold between the 1770s and 1831. Asa Briggs in *Victorian Cities* (1968) quotes a visitor from Rotherham in 1808.

The town is abominably filthy, the steam engine is pestiferous; the Dyehouses noisome and offensive, and the water of the river is as black as ink.

Thirty years later the Frenchman Alexis de Toqueville visited the city. In his *Journeys to England and Ireland* he described his visit in July 1835:

The view of Manchester from the train in 1844. Note the cows in the foreground.

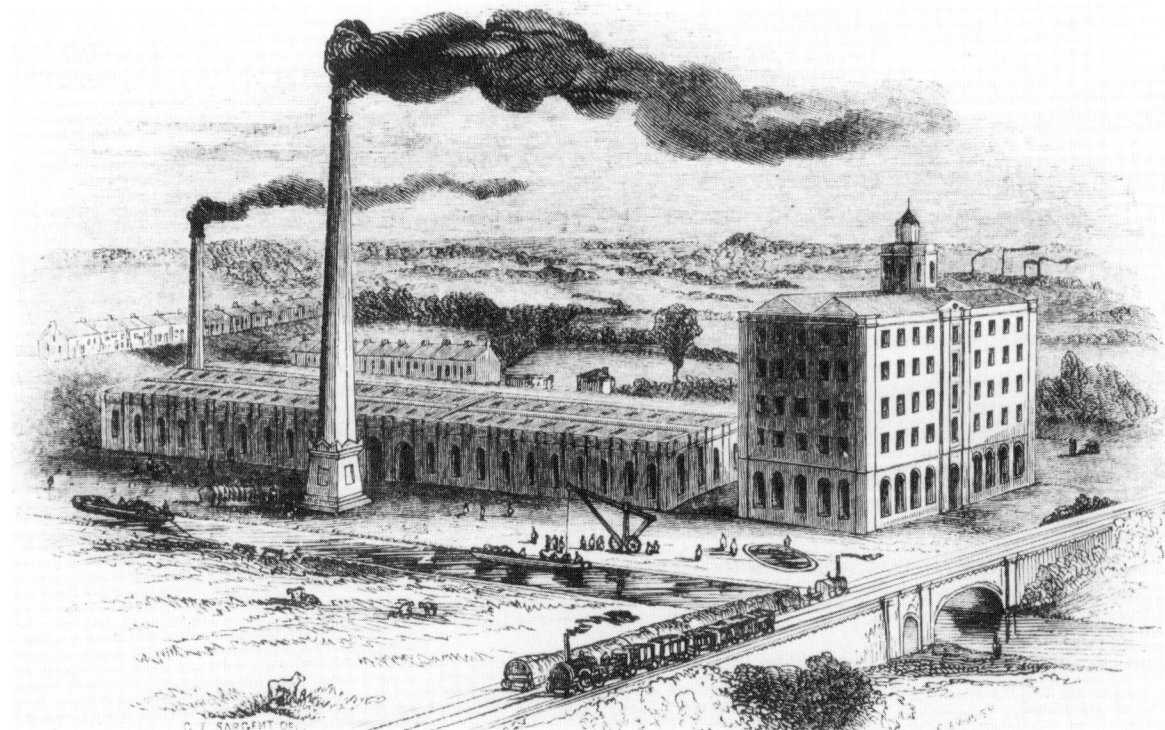

The River Irwell at Manchester (c.1850). What ▷ impression would this illustration have made upon a country visitor?

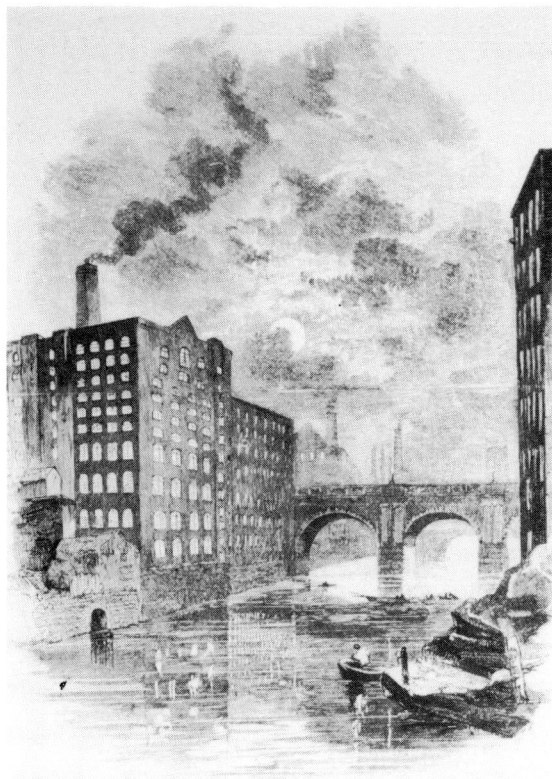

An undulating plain, or rather a collection of little hills. Below the hills, a narrow river [the Irwell], which flows to the Irish Sea. Two streams [the Medlock and the Irk] wind through the uneven ground and after a thousand bends, flow into the river.

Thirty or forty factories rise on the tops of the hills. The wretched dwellings of the poor are scattered haphazard around them . . . on ground below the level of the river and over-shadowed on every side by immense workshops, stretch marshy land which widely spaced ditches can neither drown nor cleanse.

. . . The fetid [stinking] muddy waters, stained with a thousand colours by the factories they pass . . . wander slowly round this refuge of poverty.

A sort of black smoke covers the city. The sun that shines through it is a disc without rays. Under this half daylight 300,000 human beings are ceaselessly at work.

Why did people live in such conditions and why were others keen to join them?

HOUSING IN LEEDS

Sewerage engineer Veitch gave the following evidence to the Royal Commission on the State of Large Towns in Populous Districts in 1844:

It is to be regretted that, on so great an extent of low ground destined so soon to be covered with population, some general plan of new streets should not be adopted in conformity with good drainage and ventilation.

Why were drainage and ventilation so important?

LACK OF OPEN SPACE

Dr Hawkins gave evidence to the Factory Commissioners in 1833:

It is impossible not to notice the total absence of public gardens, parks and walks at Manchester; it is scarcely in the power of the factory workmen to taste the breath of nature or to look upon its verdure [green], and this defect is a strong impediment to convalescence from disease which is usually tedious and difficult.

Mr Aston in *Picture of Manchester*, published in 1810, suggested why there were few open spaces:

. . . too minutely directed to the value of land to sacrifice much to public convenience or the conservation of health.

Do you agree with his argument?

The Slums

Each town or city had an area where the poorest and often the newest arrivals congregated. Here houses were subdivided and every room and cellar occupied. Usually these were the areas where the foul-smelling trades such as tanning, tallow-chandling and soap-making were practised.

WHAT IS A SLUM?

Roberts Williams in *London Rookeries and Colliers' Slums*, published in 1893, defined a slum:

> It may be one house but it generally is a cluster of houses, or blocks of dwellings, not necessarily dilapidated, or badly drained, or old, but usually all this and small-roomed, and, further, so hemmed in by other houses, so wanting in light and air, and therefore cleanliness, as to be wholly unfit for human habitation.

A LONDON SLUM

The *Report of the Commission of Health and Sanitary Improvement of St James, Westminster*, published in 1848, described a central London street:

> Although there is a sewer, the houses are not drained into it but into cesspools in surrounding premises. The rooms are crammed with occupants [and] are most horribly dirty, as is also the scanty furniture . . . . The cistern or water butts are NEVER cleaned out . . . the houses are let and underlet 2, 3, 4 times deep, and the privies are so filthily dirty on floors and seats as to prohibit their natural use and at the south end of the street are large premises filled with cows on the basement and upper floors, from which the stench at times is unendurable.

List the health problems which are recounted here.

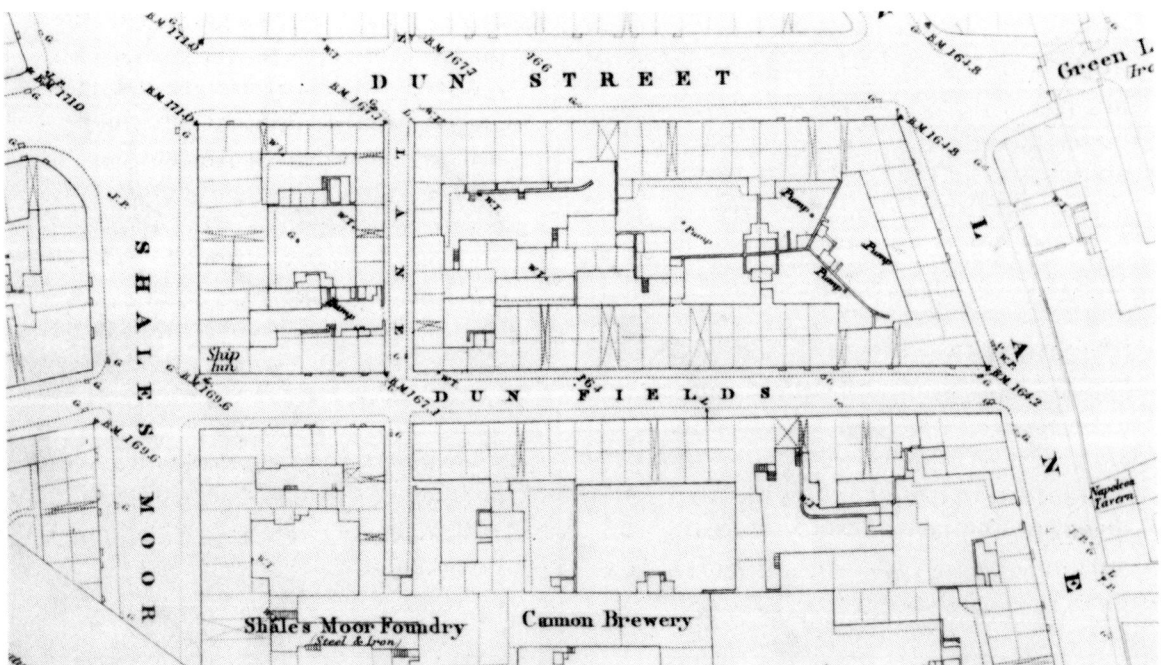

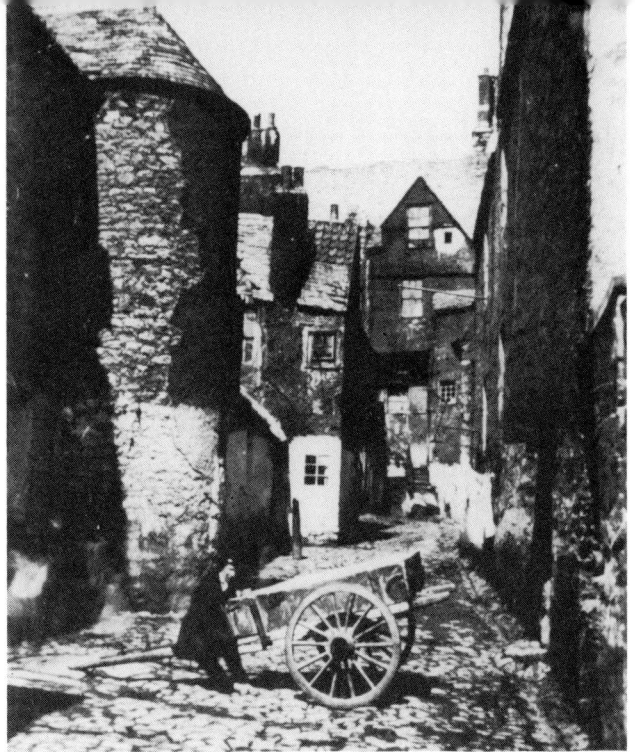

High Close, Edinburgh. The buildings were old even ▷ in 1856 when the photograph was taken. Note the drain alongside the houses on the right.

THE BITTER CRY

In 1883 *The Bitter Cry of Outcast London* was published as an anonymous, 20-page pamphlet. It is attributed to W.C. Mearns, Secretary of the London Congregational Union. Here he describes Colliers' Rents, Bermondsey:

> **To get into them you have to penetrate courts reeking with poisonous malodorous [foul-smelling] gases arising from accumulation of sewage and refuse scattered in all directions . . . you have to grope your way along dark and filthy passages swarming with vermin. Then, if you are not driven back by the intolerable stench, you may gain admittance to the dens in which these thousands of beings . . . herd together.**

Can you guess Mearns' purpose in writing the pamphlet? He then proceeded to describe the neighbourhood:

> **Reeking courts, crowded public houses, low lodging houses, and numerous brothels are to be found all around. Even the cellars are tenanted; poverty, rags, and dirt everywhere. The air is laden with disease-breeding gases. The missionaries who labour here are constantly being attacked by some malady or other . . .**

Can you identify where the slums might have been in your town?

◁ *Part of Sheffield as shown on the 25-inches-to-the-mile Ordnance Survey Map of 1853. Note the back-to-back houses, the pumps and the crosses which denote covered ways into the Courts.*

A CONTRARY VIEW

The Medical Officer of Health for Clerkenwell in his *Twenty-eighth Annual Report* of 1883 had little sympathy for the poor:

> **When these poorer people, especially the labourers, enter a house, at once begins a course of dirt and destruction . . . . The locks and handles of doors became toys for the children, and are soon demolished. The drain taps are sold at the bone and bottle shows . . . the closets are stopped up and the pans are broken. The chimneys are never swept, so that the rooms become blackened and disfigured. The paper is torn off the walls; the floor passages are never washed . . . . The very hand-rails of the staircases are broken away . . . . The windows are constantly broken and stopped up with brown paper.**

Where do your sympathies lie? With Mearns, who blames poverty for the conditions, or with the Medical Officer, who believes that the poor were responsible for the slums in which they lived?

Cellar Dwellings and Lodging Houses

The poor sought accommodation where they could find it. Closeness to work, or hope of it, and a cheap rent were essential requirements. Few of these people had regular work and so they were constantly moving on. Many properties were rented out by the room, including the attics and cellars.

NEW HOUSES IN MANCHESTER

Not all poor housing was old. Here Nassau Senior describes badly built houses in the early 1840s. Friedrich Engels quoted him in *Conditions of the Working Class in England*, published in 1844.

> I was only amazed that it is possible to maintain a reasonable state of health in such homes. [They] have been erected with the utmost disregard of everything except the immediate advantage of the speculative builder. A carpenter or builder unite to buy a series of building sites [i.e. they lease them for a number of years] and cover them with so called houses. In one place we found a whole street following the course of a ditch, because in this way deeper cellars could be secured without the cost of digging, not for storing wares or rubbish, but for dwellings of human beings. Not one house of this street escaped cholera. In general the streets of these suburbs are unpaved, with a dunghill or ditch in the middle; the houses are back to back, without ventilation and drainage, and whole families are limited to a corner of a cellar or a garret.

What was the major health hazard of these buildings?

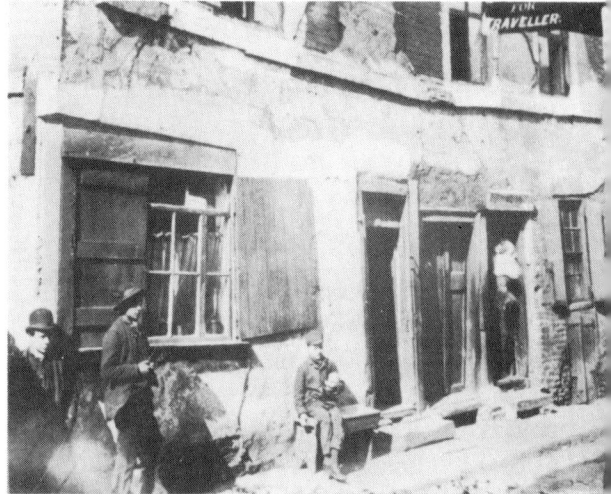

Middle Row, Croydon, Surrey c.1890. What two purposes do you think the shutters served? In 1884 a council committee was formed to consider the demolition of the worst of Middle Row (see pages 40-1).

A CELLAR DWELLING

This description comes from *Notes on Old Edinburgh*, published in 1869, by Isabella Bird.

> We entered the first room by descending two steps. It seemed to be an old coal-cellar, with an earthen floor, shining in many places from damp, and from a greenish ooze which drained through the wall from a noxious collection of garbage outside, upon which a small window could have looked had it not been filled up with brown paper and rags. The roof was unceiled, the walls were rough and broken, the only light came in from the open door, which let in unwholesome smells and sounds. No cow or horse could thrive in such a hole. It was abominable. It measured eleven feet by six feet, and the rent was 10d. per week,

THE LODGING HOUSE

These were used by both men and women who bought shelter for the night. J.M. Weylland in *These Fifty Years* (of the London City Mission) published in 1884, gave this description:

> There are many common lodging houses – when I first visited these houses, both male and female, married and unmarried, of all ages, lodged and

> paid in advance. It was nearly dark at noon, even with the door open; but as my eyes became accustomed to the dimness, I saw that the pleshings [furnishings] consisted of an old bed, a barrel with a flagstone on the top of it for a table, a three legged stool, and an iron pot.

Put yourself in the situation of a child living in the cellar. Describe your feelings on waking one winter morning.

Edwin Chadwick in *The Report on the Sanitary Conditions of the Labouring Population* (1842) believed:

> More filth, physical suffering and more disorder than Howard [a prison reformer] describes as affecting the prisoners, are to be found among the cellar population of the working people of Liverpool, Manchester, or Leeds and in large portions of the Metropolis [London].

Before this report there had been little interest in how the poor were housed. Chadwick made the clear link between bad housing and disease, and from this time bad housing became a part of the public health problems.

> slept in one room, without shame. The rooms were, very many of them, dark and filthy.

In 1851 Lord Shaftesbury was responsible for the Common Lodgings Act, which placed the lodging houses under the supervision of the police; the numbers in each were limited and the sexes separated. Whilst some improvements resulted all was not well, as Montague Williams found when he visited Mill Lane, Deptford in the 1890s:

> Here and there, written in legible characters on the outside of a building are the words, "Registered lodging house" . . . there is no adequate supervision over them . . . . At present the authorities have no power over the owner . . . . The business is sufficiently profitable to enable them to laugh at the law. For conducting his house improperly, he should, in my opinion, be liable to a fine of, say, one hundred pounds. (Montague Williams, *Round London*, 1894)

Why is Williams suggesting such a large fine?

GLASGOW LODGING HOUSES

Glasgow was no better, as the *Sanitary Journal* of 1878 reported:

> . . . the state of the lodging houses and the cellars especially, beggars [goes beyond] description; the floors thereof being packed at night with human beings – men, women and children like so many bundles of rags, and the walls and the roof black with vermin.

Compare these descriptions with those of Croydon on pages 40-1.

Overcrowding and Public Health

In his diary entry for 18 September, 1814 Herr Escher, a Swiss visitor, wrote:

> In the Old Town are to be found not only good streets and fine buildings but also the most wretched dwellings and churches that I have seen anywhere. In one house I counted no less than ten floors one piled on top of the other and there are some disgusting alleyways and horrid nooks and crannies.

What would be the particular problems of living in an old ten-storey block such as this?

OVERCROWDING IN CELLARS

Andrew Mearns in *The Bitter Cry of Outcast London* (1883) described cellar dwellers:

> Every room in these rotting and reeking tenements houses a family, often two. In one cellar, a sanitary inspector reports finding a father, mother, children, and four pigs! In another room a missionary found a man ill with smallpox, his wife just recovering from her eighth confinement, and the children running about half naked and covered with dirt. Here are seven people living in one underground kitchen and a little child lying dead in one room . . .

Later Mearns described how the occupations made the conditions worse:

> Here you are choked as you enter by the air laden with particles of the superfluous [unwanted] fur pulled

Whilst various Acts were passed during the nineteenth century the problems of the poor continued, basically because there were not enough houses or rooms at rents which they could afford. (An Enquiry of 1885 revealed that nearly half the working class paid between a quarter and a half of their income in rent.) Add to this the rapidly increasing population of the towns and the demolition of housing (often the worst) for town improvements, such as road-widening, stations, town halls, and you can see why the problem remained well into the twentieth century.

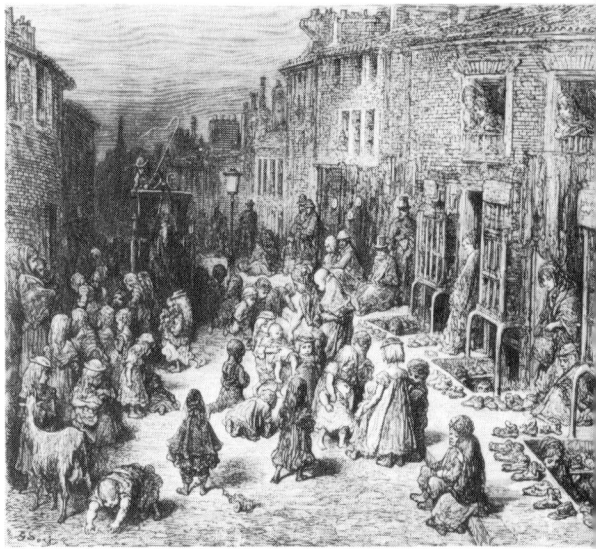

> from the skins of rabbits, rats, dogs and other animals in preparation for the farrier. Here the smell of paste and of drying match boxes:– or it may be the fragrance of stall fish and vegetables, not sold on the previous day, and kept in the room overnight.

Why were these trades carried on at home? Can you think of others which would have endangered health?

THE 1891 CENSUS

The census of 1891 required information on numbers per room and the evidence confirmed what many had feared:

$1/10$ of the total population lived more than 2 per room

$1/5$ of the population of London, Bradford and Huddersfield lived more than 2 per room

$1/4$ of the population of Plymouth lived more than 2 per room

$1/3$ of the population of the N.E. Coast lived more than 2 per room.

Check in the library to see what the figures were in your area.

◁ *Dudley Street, Seven Dials, London taken from Gustave Doré's* London *of 1872. Note how the cellars are used as shops. What impressed Doré most about this street?*

WHERE WOULD THEY GO?

The link between overcrowding and disease was clear, but if people were displaced where would they go? This problem was expressed by the Medical Officer of Health for St Marylebone, London, in *The Charity Organisation Reporter* of March 1874:

> My first impulse was to declare the house unfit for human habitation, and, by means of a magistrate's order, to remove the inmates at once. A moment's reflection, however, convinced me that by adopting that course I should really accomplish no good object, inasmuch as the poor people, thus suddenly ejected, would be compelled to seek shelter in dwellings probably more crowded or in an equally bad sanitary condition.

How could this problem be solved?

OVERCROWDING AND PUBLIC HEALTH

In 1858 the Medical Officer of Health of the Strand in London told his Vestry that even if various improvements were made problems would still remain.

> ... so long as twenty, thirty, or even forty individuals are permitted – it might almost be said, compelled – to reside in houses originally built for the accommodation of a single family, or at the most two families ...

Dr. Buchanan, the Medical Officer of Health for St Giles, London, said in his first report to his Vestry in 1857:

> If you were asked to name a single condition which shall produce an excess of zymotic diseases, an excess of consumption and lung cases, and a large infant mortality, the answer is ready and inevitable. You may produce all these diseases with most certainty ... if you will only crowd your population together so that they shall breathe sufficiently impure air.

Sewage and Refuse Disposal

A Commission of Sewers had been formed in London in the sixteenth century, but sewers were only to be used for the drainage of surface water. Another problem was that there was no central system of sewers in our cities until late in the nineteenth century. Until then there were various sewer companies whose main purpose was to provide flood protection.

IPSWICH IN 1848

In 1848 Mr Austin, the civil engineer to the town, wrote:

> Practically Ipswich was without any system of sewerage. Of sewers for the accommodation of the drainage of houses there was none; they either drain to cesspools and dead wells or not at all. The slops and refuse being thrown into the streets and the foundation of the town saturated with foul and pestilential soil.

What do you think dead wells were?

GUANO USED FOR FERTILIZER

In the late 1840s guano began to be imported from South America to be used as fertilizer. T. Fresh, the Liverpool Inspector of Nuisances, recounted how in 1851 this made the problem worse for the ordinary person:

> Prior to the introduction of guano into the country . . . the nightmen in Liverpool, not only emptied many of the middens [refuse tips] free of expense, but occasionally gave an equivalent for the privilege of doing so. [Now] the nightmen refuse to discharge any middens unless *they* were paid for doing so.

CHADWICK'S COMMENTS

On the 20 August 1848 Edwin Chadwick wrote to Lord Morpeth, the government minister who introduced the Public Health Bill in that year.

> Cesspools may be emptied, but stinking dust heaps are left, because the scavenger removes them when it suits his convenience . . . . By a fortunate concurrence the night soil, coal ashes and the dung may be removed and the court would smell sweet but for some dead cats, or a dead dog, or fish garbage, which the dustmen and sewer men under some contract decide it is not "their place" to remove.

Look at the next extract and decide why the scavengers were so selective.

Flushing the Sewers, from Henry Mayhew's London Labour and the London Poor *(1851). What dangers would the men be subject to?*

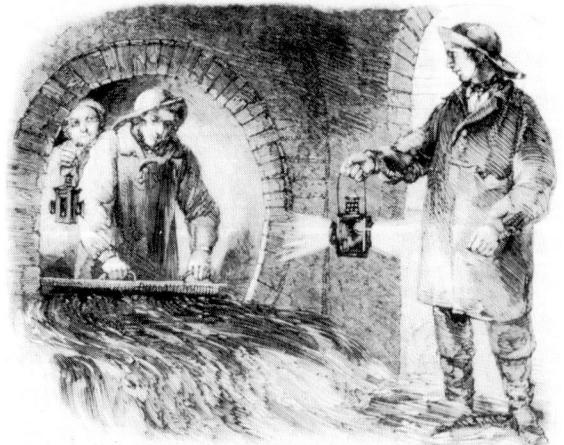

THE METROPOLITAN COMMISSION OF SEWERS

The Metropolitan Sewers Act of 1848 required that every new house built must be drained into a sewer and not into a cesspool. The Act also ended all old sewer companies and established the Metropolitan Commission of Sewers for London. Sadly, it was not up to its task and charged high rates for little return. The Lambeth Vestry Minutes of 2 August 1849 registered a common complaint:

> **Notwithstanding the defects of sewers and drains, that the filth of privies are allowed to be pumped into the sewers impregnating the air with deleterious [harmful] odours, which filth runs into the River Thames near where the water works supply the water drunk and consumed by the inhabitants.**

PUMPING STATIONS

The answer to the pollution of rivers was met by the pumping of sewage downstream, or well away from urban areas. John Deprose in *Some Accounts of the Parish of St. Clement Danes*, published in 1868, explained how London was catered for:

> **As regards the sewage of the Metropolis, now carried by a main drainage scheme far down the Thames, to the great purification of the river in London, it was found necessary to raise the whole from a lower to a higher level in the course of twelve miles through which the main drain runs. For this purpose there are two pumping stations on the North side and two on the South side of the Thames.**
>
> **Of these on the South side, one is situated in Deptford Creek . . . and the other at Crossness outfall . . . that just opened on the North side at Abbey Mills is of 1140 horse power; the latter was opened by the Prince of Wales in April 1865.**

Why could a similar system not have been introduced earlier in the century?

Where are your nearest sewage works? Note that with more scientific methods water can now be filtered and then recycled several times without damage to health.

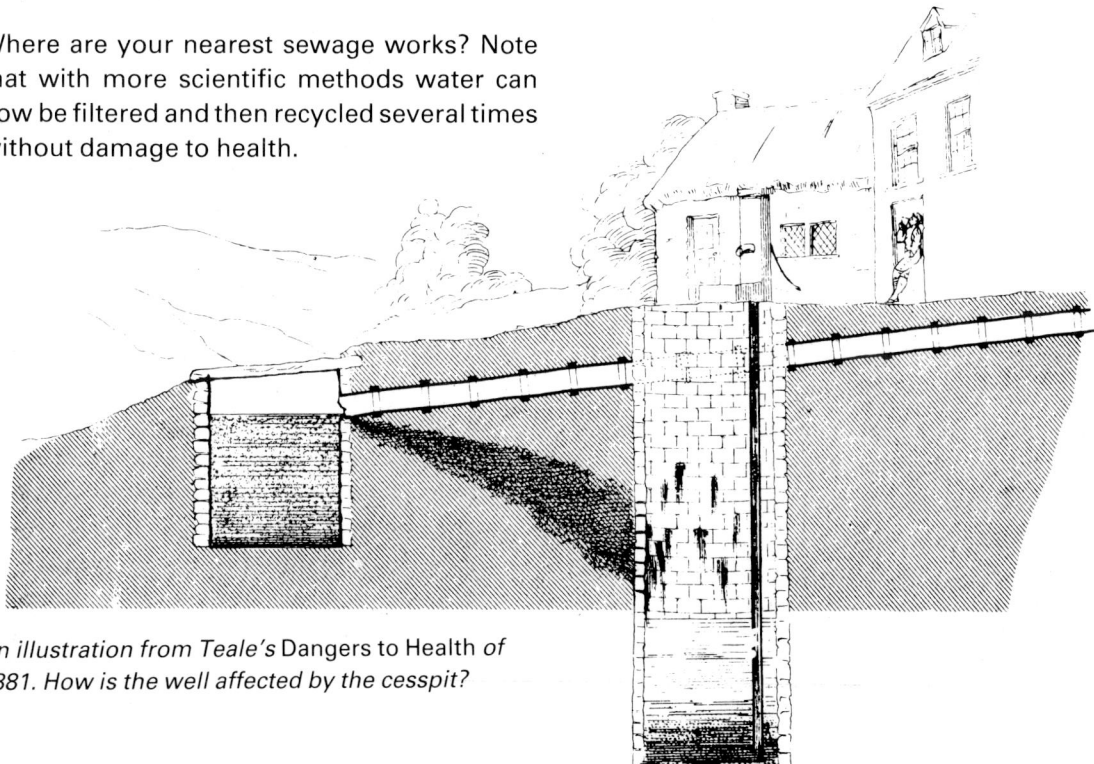

An illustration from Teale's Dangers to Health *of 1881. How is the well affected by the cesspit?*

River Pollution

Many towns drew their drinking water from nearby rivers and emptied their refuse into them. When the towns were small this was possible but with growing populations and industry it became increasingly dangerous. Factories were usually sited near rivers because water was needed for many industrial purposes and was pumped back after use full of chemical pollutants.

THE RIVER AIRE

The Leeds Intelligencer on 21 August 1841 carried an article by a civil engineer:

It [the river] is charged with the contents of about 200 W.C.s and similar places, a great number of common drains, the draining from dung hills, the Infirmary (dead leeches, poultices for patients, etc.) slaughter houses, chemicals, soap, gas, dung, dyehouses, manufactories, spent blue and black dye, pig manure, old wire wash, with all sorts of decomposed animal and vegetable substances . . . amounting to about 30,000 gallons a year of the mass of filth with which the river is loaded.

What effects must this have had upon the river?

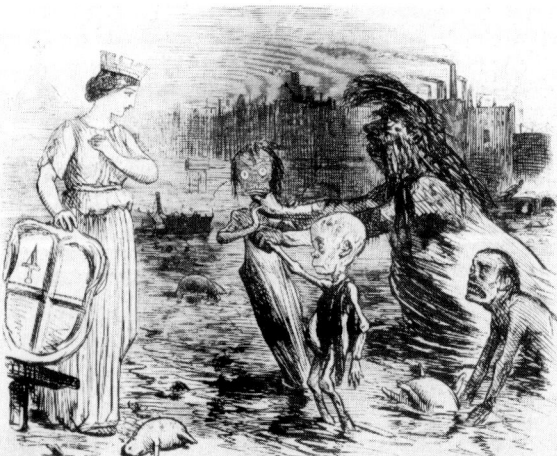

FATHER THAMES INTRODUCING HIS OFFSPRING TO THE FAIR CITY OF LONDON.
(A Design for a Fresco in the New Houses of Parliament)

THE RIVER STINK

In Bradford the canal was polluted. The Board of Surveyors described it in 1843:

The drains of the town are emptied into the watercourse, and principally above the flood gates. Besides, on both sides of the stream there are a great many factories of various kinds of manufacture, etc., the soil, refuse and filth of which falls into the beck. In summer-time the water is low, and all the filth accumulates for weeks, or months, above the floodgates, and emits a most offensive smell. This noxious compound is conveyed through the sluice gates into the canal.

It is not surprising that the Health of Towns Commission described Bradford in 1844 as "the dirtiest, filthiest, and worst regulated town in the Kingdom".

THE THAMES

As the population of London grew the pollution of the Thames increased. Chadwick's belief that the sewers should be flushed into the Thames did not help and 209 public sewers discharged into it. The Educational Review of 1850 described the problem:

The refuse and the dirt from two million individuals . . . the enormous accumulation of waste and dead animal and vegetable matter . . . the blood and offal of the slaughter-houses, – the outpourings from the Gas Works, dye-works, breweries, distilleries, glue-works, bone-works, tanneries,

A Punch cartoon of 1858. What message is the cartoonist conveying to his readers?

Manchester had three rivers: the Irwell and its tributaries, the Medlock and the Irk. The Irwell divided Manchester from Salford. The anonymous author of a *Pictorial History of Lancashire*, published in 1844, described this river:

> **The river is really unsightly. Gas drainings, the refuse of factories, unite with countless other abominations to contaminate the stream, and render it equally fatal to animal and vegetable life.**

He then went on to describe the Medlock:

> **The aspect of the Medlock is still worse, – as seen from the bridge leading into Chorlton, it is nothing but an overgrown puddle. It is however unfair to judge of these rivers in their artificial state. The Upper Vale of the Medlock offers a most tempting view . . . . If we cross the bridge and visit the crescent of Salford, we shall see a delightful view, exhibiting what the Irwell might have been had its waters not been enslaved to cotton.**

> **chemical and other works, and a thousand nameless pollutions; – all find their way into the Thames. The mixture is next washed backwards and forwards by the tide; and having been thoroughly stirred up and finely commuted by the unceasing splash of 298 steam-boats, is then pumped up for the wealthiest cup in the world!**

What made it worse was that half the population south of the river received their water from the Thames and only the minority of water companies sought to filter the water.

The Irk fared no better. Dr Kay, local doctor and member of Manchester's Board of Health, described the Irk Valley and the mass of cottages

> **. . . filling the insalubrious [unhealthy] valley through which the Irk flows. [The Irk] receives excrementitious matter from some sewers in this portion of the town – the drainage from the Gas Works, and filth of the most pernicious character from bone works, tanneries, size [paste] manufactories . . .** (*The Moral and Physical Condition of the Working Class Employed in Cotton Manufacture in Manchester*, 1832)

List the ways in which these three rivers were polluted.

Today our rivers are much cleaner. Try and find out why this is so.

Factories at the Kelham Island Weir on the River Don, Sheffield. Compare this modern photograph with the one of the Irwell in the first section.

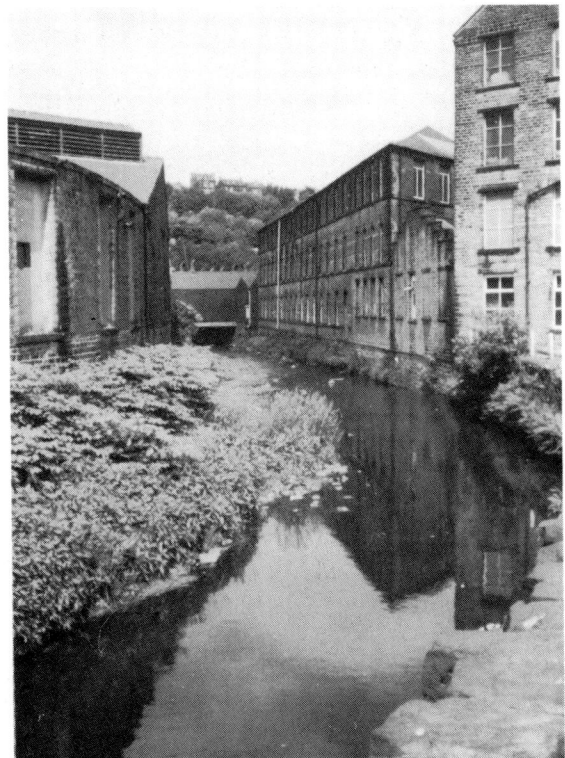

Air Pollution

In the nineteenth century there was a view commonly held that dirt and grime were a necessary price to pay for industry, wealth and jobs. The Northern saying "Where there's muck there's brass" expresses this view. In the early part of the century there were no regulations about smoke pollution, just as there were no restrictions on building.

A FOREIGN VIEW

J.G. May was a German visitor to Britain. This extract from his diary of 1814 describes the West Midlands:

> Wolverhampton in Staffordshire has many ironworks and it is famed for the manufacture of locks of all kinds. The whole district between Wolverhampton and Birmingham is covered with coal pits and ironworks. Steam engines are to be seen all over the place. The fields are covered with soot and the air is polluted with smoke so that little can grow in this area. It is hard to find a green leaf on the trees and hedges. Some parts of the district look as if they were suffering from a destructive fire.

Is May describing an industrial town or the countryside?

MANCHESTER OBSERVED

Hans Casper Escher, a Swiss architect and founder of an engineering firm, described his first view of Manchester in his diary entry for 20 August 1814:

> In Manchester there is no sun and no dust. Here there is always a dense cloud of smoke to cover the sun while the light rain – which seldom lasts all day – turns the dust into a fine paste.

Why would a Swiss have been particulary shocked by Manchester?

By the time the author of the *Pictorial History of Lancashire* visited the city in 1845 industry had increased, as had the population. He described the view:

Manchester from the London and North-Western Railway (c. 1854). Compare this print with the written descriptions in this section.

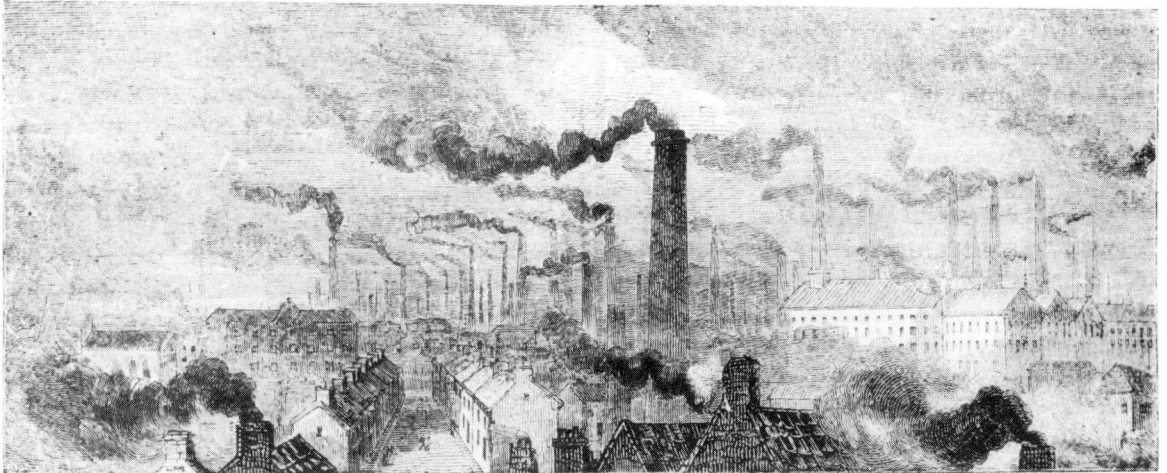

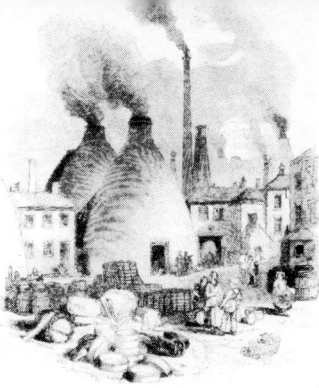

A pottery kiln in Staffordshire (c.1854) Why may the smoke from the kilns have been more dangerous than those from the factory chimneys?

The prospect is anything but cheering. Forests of chimneys, clouds of smoke and volumes of vapour, like the seething of some stupendous cauldron, occupy the entire landscape; there is no sky, but a dark gray haze, variegated by masses of smoke more dense than the rest, which look like fleeces of black wool, or clouds of subliminated [raised] ink.

Imagine that you are a recent arrival in Manchester from a small village in Ireland. Describe your first impressions.

THE NOVELISTS' VIEW

There follow two descriptions of industrial towns. What have they in common, and in what ways do they differ from the earlier descriptions?

Coketown

Charles Dickens travelled to Preston in 1854 to collect material for *Hard Times*. Coketown in the novel is probably based on his experiences there.

It was a town of red brick, or of brick that would have been red if the smoke and ashes had allowed it . . . . It was a town of machinery and tall chimneys, out of which interminable serpents of smoke trailed themselves for ever and ever, and never got uncoiled.

LONDON FOG

Thomas Miller, writing in *Picturesque Sketches of London* in 1852, described the London fog:

You fancy that all the smoke which had ascended for years from the thousands of London chimneys had fallen down all at once, after having rotted somewhere above the clouds, smelling as if it had been kept too long, and making you wheeze as if all the colds in the world were rushing into your head for warmth, and did not care a straw about killing a few thousands of people, as long as they could but lodge comfortably for a few hours anywhere.

Why was fog such a hazard to health? Try and find out how the Clean Air Acts have cleared our cities of these dangerous fogs.

Milton

Elizabeth Gaskell described the approach to a Northern industrial town in her novel *North and South*. It was first published in 1854, and she called her town Milton.

For several miles before they reached Milton, they saw a deep lead-covered cloud hanging over the horizon in the direction in which it lay. It was all the darker from contrast with the pale gray-blue of the country sky. Nearer to the town the air had a faint taste of smell and smoke . . . . Here and there a great oblong many-windowed factory stood up, like a hen among her chickens, puffing out black unparliamentary smoke.

N.B. Under an Act of 1847 every chimney constructed *after* that date had to consume its own smoke.

The Burial of the Dead

Nothing better illustrates the relationship between public health, overcrowding and the rapid expansion of our towns than the problems of the dying and the dead.

THE DEAD AMONGST THE LIVING

Edwin Chadwick in a *Report on the Practice of Interment in Towns*, published in 1843, included the evidence of Mr Leonard, surgeon and Medical Officer of St Martin's in the Fields, London:

> There are some houses in my district that have from 45 to 60 persons of all ages under one roof, and in the event of death, the body often occupies the only bed till they raise the money to pay for a coffin, which is often several days . . .

> Upon the 2nd of February, 1843 H ——————— , in Heathcock Court, died of fever. I recommended the immediate removal of the body from the attic room of small dimensions, but it was retained about ten days, the widow not consenting to have it buried by the parish, and not being able to collect funds sooner, their only child was seized with fever, and was several weeks ill.

What would be the health risks of leaving a dead body in a room with the living?

What remains of St Alphage's graveyard, Greenwich. Note how the older headstones have been removed to the sides. The graveyard is no longer used for burials.

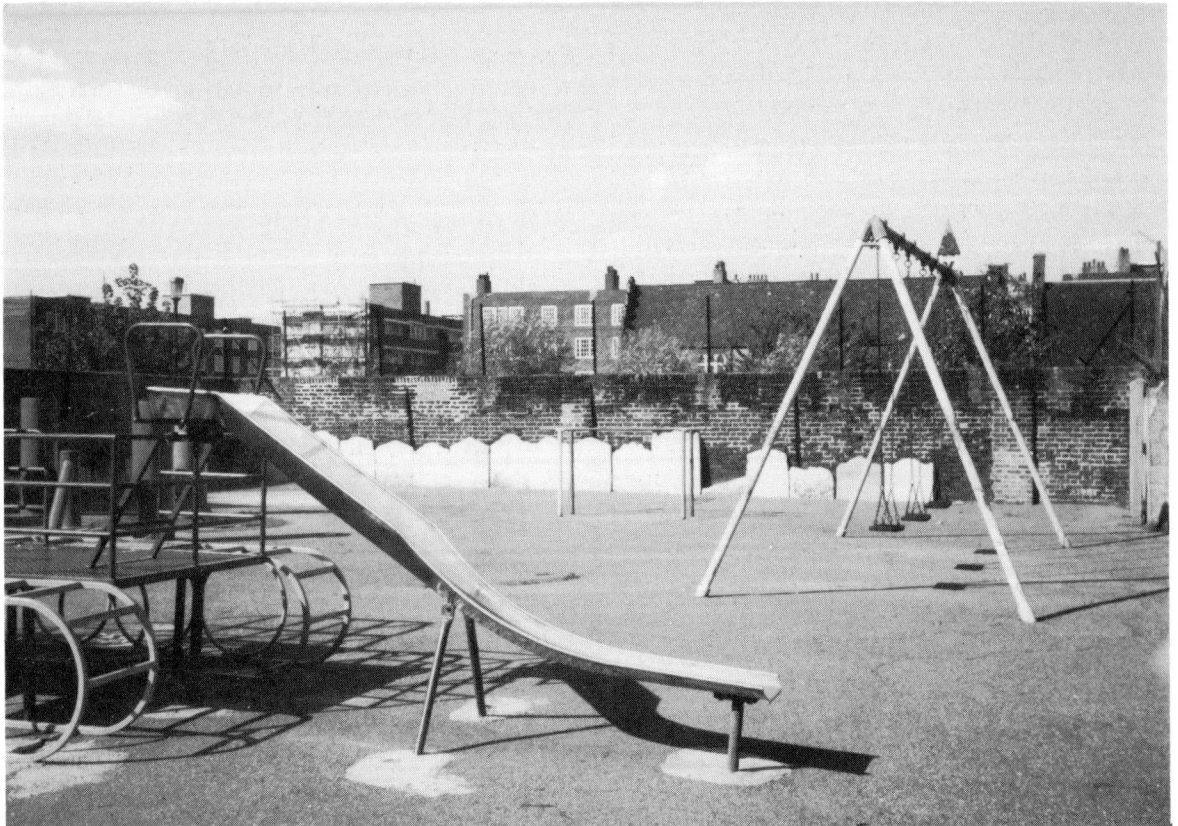

A DERELICT GRAVEYARD

The Medical Officer of St George's District of Manchester wrote to Lord Shaftesbury on 1 November 1866, complaining about the scandalous conditions of the abandoned parish burial ground which was now surrounded by housing.

> **Occasionally a human skull is turned up and thrown about; more than forty thousand dead lay there, yet not a gravestone is left; some may be found forming part of the floor of cottages, others may be seen placed in privies.**

A sure sign that a graveyard has been reorganized is when the head-stones are placed around the surrounding wall.

THE PORTUGAL STREET BURIAL GROUND

Henry Besant included in his *London in the Nineteenth Century* (1909) various reports on the state of the London burial grounds in the late 1830s:

> **The Portugal Street ground is truly shocking. On the testimony of two professors of King's College, who examined it to see if planting trees were practicable, it is crammed with coffins no less than two feet, in some places fifteen inches, below the surface, and yet "the work goes on". The dreadful practice . . . has been exposed half a dozen times . . . . They are obliged to put up "coping boards", on the side of a grave, to prevent the public seeing the "work", before the digger is in to his knees. This, however, does not save the inhabitants from overlooking houses in Clement's Lane, who make dreadful complaints, in addition to which, fever, *"The Pestilence that Walketh in Darkness"*, broods over the miserable place.**

Why did this burial ground present a health hazard?

INNER CITY GRAVEYARDS

In Thomas Miller's *Picturesque Sketches of London* (1852) he outlined the problem for London and other rapidly growing cities:

> **When our old churches were first built, they stood in wide, open, breezy places, – such was Bartholomew Church, when Smithfield was really a field . . . we have hemmed in the spots with streets and tall warehouses, until they have become so close and breathless, that even the sparrows forsake their "old ancestral eaves" and seek for other roosting places.**

Look at a late nineteenth-century map and see whether your parish church was surrounded by buildings.

IMPROVEMENTS

The government's response in London and elsewhere in the late 1830s was to allow commerical cemeteries in the surrounding suburbs. However by 1850 in London many of these were nearly full and there was a demand for public cemeteries. Examples of the old and new can be seen in J. Wilson's *Gazeteer of England and Wales* (1876):

> #### Manchester
>
> **The Rusholme Road cemetery, in Charlton-cum-Medlock, was opened in 1821; was then surrounded by green fields, giving it a rural aspect, became surrounded before 1857 by brick buildings . . . and was closed.**
>
> **. . . The General Cemetery, in Rochdale Road, about 2 miles from the City, occupies about 11 acres.**

Cholera

Cholera came to Britain on various occasions in the nineteenth century: in 1831-2, 1848-9, 1853-4, 1865-6 and 1893. Its symptoms were horrific – violent stomach pains, vomitting and diarrhoea. The victim's skin turned blue and he had great difficulty in breathing. His chance of recovery was only 50 per cent.

THE CHOLERA'S COMING

These verses were written during the first outbreak in 1831-2 when trade was bad and people were hungry:

> The cholera's coming, oh dear, oh dear,
> The cholera's coming, oh dear!
> To prevent hunger's call
> A kind of pest from Bengal
> Has come to feed all
> With the cholera, dear.
>
> The people are starving, oh dear, oh dear,
> The people are starving, oh dear,
> If they don't quickly hop
> To the parish soup shop
> They'll go off with a pop
> From the cholera, dear.

Cholera had spread from India and was sometimes called Asian Cholera. What does the writer believe causes cholera?

CHOLERA STRIKES QUICKLY

Charles Greville in his journal for 25 July 1832 recorded:

> Mrs. Smith young and beautiful . . . (who) dressed to go to church on Sunday morning when she was seized with the disorder and died at 11 at night.

In that year some 18,000 people died from the disease.

CHOLERA IN WHITECHAPEL

Cholera returned in 1848-9. There were many theories as to its cause. Chadwick made the clear link with dirt, miasma (smell) and polluted water and thus good was often done without real understanding. The General Board of Health's Report of 1850 described Christopher Court, Rosemary Lane, London:

> The court is a cul-de-sac; the entrance is narrow, and covered over by the houses in Rosemary Lane, at the upper end is a large dust hole, full of filth of every description . . . on the first floor of one house, 8 cases of cholera, of which 3 were fatal; the door at the foot of the stairs was shut, and on opening it I was repeatedly driven back by the horrid odour and stench of a privy downstairs. This was one of the dirtiest places which human beings ever visited . . . not a breath of fresh air reached them, all was abominable. After getting upstairs my head reeked in the sickening atmosphere, and on reaching the top, and surrounded by the dead and the dying, I was compelled to rush to the window and open it. I threw off the contents of my stomach, and supported myself on the miserable, rotten straw bed.

What conclusions about the causes of cholera would you draw from this account?

ate.	Sex. M. or F.	Age.	Occupation.	Residence.	Result.	Cholera, or Chol. Diarrh.
g. 6	F	32	Butcher's wife	Walton-road, St. Paul's	Death in 10 hours	C
12	F	45	Charwoman	Gas-street, St. Ebbe's	Recovery *	C
12	M	23	Prisoner	County gaol	Recovery	CD
15	F	8	Carter's daughter	Gas-street	Death, Aug. 17	CD
19	M	50	Prisoner	County gaol	Recovery, Sep. 24	CD
29	F	34	Tailor	Gas-street	Recovery, Sep. 5	C
30	M	9	Carter's son	Gas-street	Recovery, Sep. 4	C
30	M	20	Prisoner	County gaol	Recovery, Sep. 15	CD
30	F	19	Butcher's daughter	Gas-street	Recovery, Sep. 6	C
30	F	4	Soldier's daughter	Gas-street	Recovery, Sep. 6*	C
30	M	40	Labourer	Gas-street	Recovery	
30	M	30	Railway Porter	New Osney	Recovery	CD
31	M	3	Shoemaker's son	Blackfriars'-road, St. Ebbe's	Death, Aug. 31	C
p. 1	F	15 mos.	Labourer's daugh.	Gas-street	Recovery, Sep. 8*	C
1	F	40	Charwoman	Mazey's-yard, St. Ebbe's	Recovery, Sep.14*	CD
1	M	72	Labourer	Sparks's Yard, St. Aldate's	Death, Sep. 3	C
2	M	49	Pipemaker a	Waterloo Build., Blackfr.-rd.	Death, Sep. 4	C
2	M	35	Groom	George's-yd., St. Clement's	Recovery, Sep. 9	C
2	M	32	Shoemaker	Church-street, St. Ebbe's	Death, Sep. 5	C
2	M	14 mos.	†	On the River	Death, Sep. 2	C
3	F	16 mos.	Shoemaker's dau.	Blackfriars'-road	Death, Sep. 3	C
3	F	72	Servant's wife	Gas-street	Death, Sep. 4	C
4	F	63	None b	High-st., St. Peter's in East	Death, Sep. 4	CD
4	M	43	Fishmonger c	Market-street, St. Michael's	Death, Sep. 6	
4	M	48	Milkman d	Marston	Recovery, Sep. 10	C
4	M	42	Architect	St. Aldate-street	Death, Sep. 4	C
4	M	15 mos.	Carpenter's son	Godfrey's Row, St. Ebbe's	Death, Sep. 6*	C
4	F	19	Tailor	Gas-street	Recovery, Sep. 6*	C
5	M	69	Tailor	Church-street, St. Ebbe's	Death, Sep. 7	CD
5	M	5 mos.	Laundress's son e	Near the Church, St. Giles's	Death, Sep. 8	CD
5	F	45	Washerwoman	Friar's Entry, S. Mary Magd.	Recovery, Sep. 7	CD
5	F	38	Prisoner	County gaol	Death, Sep. 19	CD
5	F	40	Labourer's wife	Jericho Gardens, St. Paul's	Death, Sep. 13	C
6	M	60	Boatman	Hythe Bridge, St. Thomas	Death, Sep. 7	C
6	F	20	Labourer's wife	Mazey's-yard	Recovery, Sep. 9	C
6	F	21	Washerwoman	Blackfriars'-road	Recovery, Oct. 4*	C
6	F	4	Labourer's daugh.	Park-End-street, St.Thomas	Death, Sep. 6	C
6	M	34	Labourer	Park-End-street	Death, Sep. 6	C
7	F	55	Policeman's wife	Gas-street	Death, Sep. 8	C
7	M	33	Coal merchant f	Hythe Bridge	Recovery, Sep. 21	C
7	M	56	Surgeon g	St. Clement's Alms-house	Death, Sep. 9	C
7	F	36		St. Giles's Road West	Recovery, Sep. 18	CD
7	M	50	Mason	Friar's Wharf, St. Ebbe's	Recovery, Sep. 14	CD
7	F	28	Waiter	Cornmarket-street	Recovery, Sep. 17	C
8	F	3 mos.		Bath-street, St. Clement's	Death, Sep. 13	CD
8	F	36	Labourer's wife	Park-End-street	Death, Sep. 8	C

◁ *Part of a table listing the cholera cases in Oxford in 1854. It is taken from Henry Acland's* Memoir on the Cholera at Oxford.

SANITARY PRECAUTIONS (1883)

The Medical Officer of Health (M.O.H.) of the parish of St James and St John, Clerkenwell, London advised that precautions should be taken against

(1) **Drainage, refuse, etc.** (2) **Ventilation** (3) **Water supply** (4) **Improper food** (5) **Diarrhoea** (6) **Sinks** (7) **Disinfectants** (8) **Dustbins.**

Can you suggest what he might have recommended under each heading. He concluded with the warning:

> As cholera is prevailing abroad, and may possibly be brought here, it may well be pointed out that in former visitations, when attention has been paid to the above precautions, its advent has been harmless, but when they have been neglected severe mortality has ensued.

CHOLERA IN OXFORD, 1854

In his *Memoir on the Cholera at Oxford in the Year 1854* published in 1856, Dr Henry Wentworth Acland described one particular group of houses:

> They are described thus particularly *because* they are *not* especially bad: an overcoloured picture of wretchedness destroys the purpose of him who draws it. Many rooms in Oxford are far worse than these. There is an open street in front; a passage at the side: a yard thirty-five feet long behind: there was a privy behind not specially foul; a pump removed twenty feet from it. A privy far worse was attached to an adjoining house, and there no Diarrhoea of note occurred. There is therefore here the one condition of too many people in too small space. This is, in plain words, life in *poisoned air*.

Why does this account differ from the Whitechapel one? What does Acland believe is the chief problem?

The first to make a direct link between cholera and water was Dr John Snow in 1849, but it was not proved until 1884, when Robert Koch isolated the cholera baccillus and traced it to Bengal. Sadly, in 1861 Queen Victoria's husband, Albert, had died from the disease. Try and find whether there was a cholera epidemic in your area.

Epidemic and Infectious Diseases

The causes of many epidemic diseases were not understood until the 1860s, but the relationship between dirt and disease had been illustrated by Chadwick some 20 years before. One Sheffield report said that "the filth track, the cholera track and the fever track are identical".

TYPHOID

The water-borne diseases such as cholera and typhoid killed many people. In 1838 56,000 people died from the latter. Chadwick in the *Sanitary Condition of the Labouring Population* (1842) wrote:

> The annual slaughter in England and Wales from preventible causes of typhus which attacks persons in the vigour of life, appears to be double the amount of what was suffered by the Allied Armies at the battle of Waterloo.

Why would this make such an impact on the readers?

CERNE ABBAS, DORSET

In his report Chadwick used evidence from Poor Law unions throughout the country. Here John Fox, the medical officer of the Cerne Union, outlined the problems of the rural poor:

> Most of the cottages . . . some mere mud hovels, are situated in low, damp places . . . . In [one] a family consisting of six persons, two had fever; the mud floor of their cottage was at least one foot below the lane; it consisted of *one* small room only, in the centre of which stood a foot-ladder reaching to the edges of the platform which extended over nearly one-half of the room, and upon which were placed two beds, with space between them for one person only to stand, whilst the outside of each touched the thatch.

What were the main public health problems in this cottage?

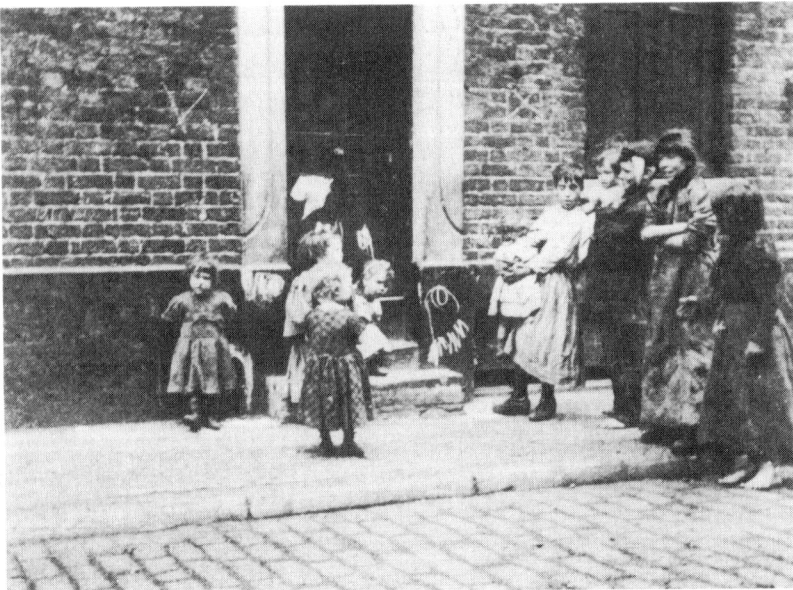

◁Waiting for an ambulance to remove a fever patient from an East End house (1899). Note the bare feet.

The distribution of deaths in ▷ certain areas of Sheffield. A report was prepared by the M.O.H. in 1877 on the application of the Artisans' Dwelling Act and presented to the Council in 1878. See the O.S. map of Sheffield on page 8 and identify the streets.

In 1842 there was a scarlet fever epidemic in Blackpool. A meeting held at the National school resolved:

> . . . the owners and occupiers of land and houses within the town [be requested] to cause all nuisances connected with their property to be removed and that their cottages be thoroughly cleaned and whitewashed.

In addition the meeting warned Mr Clifton, the largest landowner, about the

> . . . present unhealthy state of the town and respectfully requested that the large ditch which receives the wash of the town at the close gates, which, in the opinion of the medical men is highly prejudicial to the health of the inhabitants, be removed.

Why do you think that the meeting was so respectful to Mr Clifton? Clearly little was done, as a letter of 10 April 1847 from Mr Dean of South Shore, Blackpool, to Mr Clifton's agent shows:

> There seems to be sufficient cause for the fever in the want of sanitary regulations. I believe (and you can perhaps yourself by facts compared with the theory) that early in the Spring the manure heaps which lie so close to the dwellings are turned or removed and most noxious gas escapes. This is drawn through the door towards the fire and the stream of course passes through the midst of the family. Besides some houses require privys and many bedrooms are open to the shippen [cattle shed]. Can you do anything to compel the regular whitewashing of the houses quarterly or cause the dirty holes round the houses to be filled up and the manure placed at least ten yards from the doors in proper places?

Which major health problems does Mr Dean identify?

ILLNESS IN SCHOOLCHILDREN

The log books of Walton and Felixstowe National school showed the speed at which disease spread.

> Oct 12 1877   There is a great deal of sickness in the two villages. I am obliged to keep in several of the boys to do their lessons before they leave school in the afternoon, as otherwise I cannot get them done at all.
> Oct 19   The sickness [scarlet fever] has greatly increased in the village.
> Dec 14   The school continues to grow less, the illness called mumps is spreading.
> May 23 1879   The school was closed on account of a severe attack of measles in both Walton and Felixstowe, twenty families affected, and it was spreading rapidly.

Scarlet fever and measles often took the lives of schoolchildren. How are we protected today?

Streets, &c.	Zymotic Deaths.	Other Deaths.	Streets, &c.	Zymotic Deaths.	Other Deaths.
GROUP No. 1.			GROUP No. 4.		
Green street	1	4	Edward street	8	28
reet	1	0	Cornhill	1	1
ne (one side, part of)	0	0	Marsden lane	0	0
r street	0	1	Brocco street	1	3
arade	0	2	Solly street	4	25
reet	0	1	Wheeldon street	1	4
ls	4	4	Wheeldon lane	0	1
e (part of)	1	1	Kenyon street	2	3
eet (one side of)	0	10	Kenyon alley	3	1
noor	4	16	Beet street (part of)	3	16
ls	0	1	Siddall street (part of)	0	2
r square	0	1			
yard	0	0	TOTAL	23	84
TOTAL	11	41			

Chadwick and the Prevention of Disease

Edwin Chadwick had been largely responsible for the New Poor Law in 1834. Parishes were now grouped together into larger units called Poor Law unions, which not only dealt with the unemployed poor, but also the sick and old. Poor Law doctors were appointed and many workhouses had hospitals. Chadwick wrote the bulk of the 1842 *Report on Sanitary Conditions of the Labouring Population*.

LITTLE BEING DONE

Chadwick was particularly critical of lack of action on improving drainage and ventilation. The 1842 report showed clearly how little the local parishes and towns were doing to prevent disease.

> **Such is the absence of civic economy in some of our towns that their condition in respect to cleanliness is almost as bad as that of an encamped horde, or an undisciplined soldiery. The discipline of the army has advanced beyond the economy of the town . . . . The towns, whose population never change their encampment have no such care, and whilst the houses, streets, courts, lanes, and streams are polluted and rendered pestilential, the civic officers have generally contented themselves with the most barbarous expedients, or sit still amongst the pollution.**

Why does Chadwick believe that the poor in the towns are worse off than soldiers in the army? Why would a comparison with the army be so relevant at this time?

The title page of the report written by Chadwick.▷
Which part of the population did it consider? Why was it limited?

THE ARTERIAL SYSTEM

In a letter to Lord Francis Egerton written on 1 October 1845 Chadwick explained what his new system needed.

> **The carrying of water into every house, the removal of all excretion in suspension in water by means of the soil-pan, etc. . . the proof that the water-closet may be made mechanically cheaper than the cesspool.**

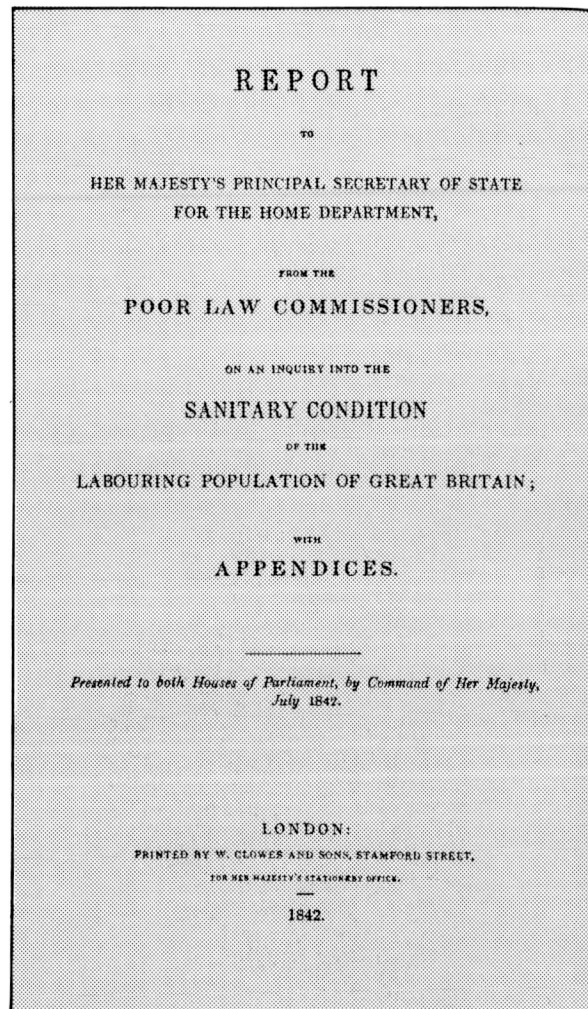

REPORT

TO

HER MAJESTY'S PRINCIPAL SECRETARY OF STATE FOR THE HOME DEPARTMENT,

FROM THE

POOR LAW COMMISSIONERS,

ON AN INQUIRY INTO THE

SANITARY CONDITION

OF THE

LABOURING POPULATION OF GREAT BRITAIN;

WITH

APPENDICES.

Presented to both Houses of Parliament, by Command of Her Majesty, July 1842.

LONDON:

PRINTED BY W. CLOWES AND SONS, STAMFORD STREET,
FOR HER MAJESTY'S STATIONERY OFFICE.

1842.

Chadwick wanted W.C.s in all houses, and a system by which they would be linked up with the sewers. This required a constant supply of water to each house, to flush the solid excreta into, and then out of, the sewers. This was what he meant by the arterial system. One loose end remained, and Chadwick referred to this in his conclusion to the 1842 Report:

> **the pollution of the water of the river into which the sewers are discharged.**

Look back and see how his system compared with the existing sanitary conditions for the poor.

CHADWICK'S CONCLUSION

One of the major conclusions of the 1842 report was

> **. . . that the expense of public drainage, of supplies of water laid on in houses, and of means of improved cleansing would be a pecuniary [financial] gain by diminishing the existing charges attendant on sickness and premature mortality.**

A new system was going to be costly. How then did Chadwick believe that a real saving would be made?

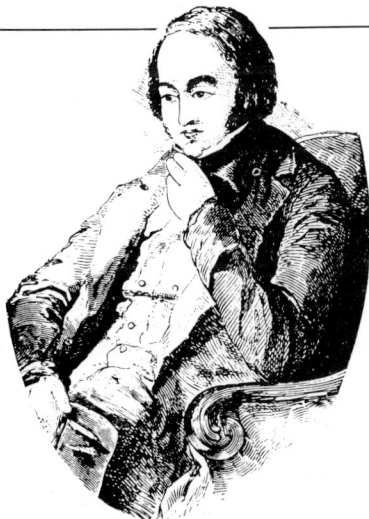

THE HEALTH OF TOWNS COMMISSION

The government was worried by some of the more radical recommendations of the report, such as the abolition of the many private water companies, so they played for time by establishing a Royal Commision. Chadwick was again the author of the report, which studied 50 major towns, one-sixth of the population. The Commission was concerned with the mechanical details of drainage and sewage and contained famous scientists and engineers, such as Brunel. Their task was often unpleasant as Chadwick indicated in a letter to Major Graham in 1843:

> **My vacation has been absorbed in visiting with Mr. Smith and Dr. Playfair the worst parts of some of the worst towns. Dr. Playfair has been knocked up by it and has been seriously ill. Mr. Smith has had a little dysentery. Sir Henry la Bêche (a geologist) was obliged at Bristol to stand up at the end of alleys and vomit while Dr. Playfair was investigating overflowing privies, Sir Henry was obliged to give it up.**

What risks did the investigators face?

CHADWICK'S ACHIEVEMENTS

Harriet Martineau in the *History of the Peace* (1858) paid tribute to Chadwick:

> **Mr. Chadwick has no doubt done more than any other man in direct furtherance of the general health.**

Do you agree?

◁ *Edwin Chadwick in 1848. He was forced into retirement in 1854, lived another 36 years, but never took another job.*

The Death Rate

LIFE CHANCES IN TOWN AND COUNTRY

One of the most revealing details of Chadwick's 1842 report was the average age of death in certain urban and rural areas. They included:

	1 Gentlemen, Professional Persons & their Families	2 Tradesmen, and their Families	3 Labourers & Artisans and their Families
Manchester	38	20	17
Bolton	34	23	18
Bethnal Green	45	26	16
Liverpool	35	22	15
Leeds	44	27	19
Kendal(Cumbria)	45	39	34
Rutland(county)	52	41	38

Why did people living in the last two areas live longer? Why did people in column 3 die so young?

THE NATIONAL DEATH RATE

Another way of looking at the progress of public health is to look at the death rate, which is calculated by giving the numbers of deaths for every 1000 people. These figures are for England and Wales

1838	22.4	1881	18.9
1841	21.6	1891	20.2
1851	22.0	1901	16.9
1861	21.6	1938	11.6
1871	22.6		

What is the major conclusion you would draw from these figures?

The quarterly death figures presented to Croydon ▷ Town Council. What is significant about the infant deaths?

In 1836 the Births, Marriages and Deaths Act was passed. This required that these were to be officially recorded. Before that time details were kept in various parish registers; now they were to be collected locally and then totalled so that, each quarter of the year, precise figures could be given for each district and also the whole country.

CORPORATION OF CROYDON.

QUARTERLY MORTALITY
OF
THE BOROUGH OF CROYDON
(CROYDON URBAN SANITARY DISTRICT),

From APRIL 1st, 1888, to JUNE 30th, 1888, both inclusive.

During the quarter ending June 30th, 1888, 645 *births* and 298 *deaths* were registered as having occurred in the Borough of Croydon.

Of the 645 births, 357 were those of males, 288 those of females. The birth-rate was 26·96 per 1,000 of the population; the average birth-rate of the corresponding quarter of the ten preceding years being 31·39 per 1,000.

The 298 deaths were at an annual rate of 12·45 per 1,000 of the population, the average rate of the corresponding quarter of the ten previous years being 15·67 per 1,000.

The following death rates for the quarter are taken from the Registrar General's Quarterly Return for the purpose of comparison:— All England and Wales, 17·50 ; the Town Districts of England and Wales. 17·70; the Country Districts, 17·20 ; London "Outer Ring' (Suburbs), 13·40 per 1,000.

Distributing the 34 deaths in the Union House and Infirmary and the 6 deaths in the Croydon General Hospital among the wards of the borough proportionally to their populations, the death-rates of the several wards per 1,000 estimated inhabitants were—West Ward 13·28, Central Ward 14·31, East Ward 6·91, South Ward 12·87, South Norwood Ward, 8·76, Upper Norwood Ward—Upper Norwood sub-division 15·83, Thornton Heath sub-division 16·72.

As regards sex, 154 were the deaths of males, 144 those of females, and the mortality among males was 14·39, and among females 10·89 per 1,000 of each sex respectively estimated to be living in the borough.

Of the total deaths from all causes, 19—or about 7 per cent.—were due to the principal zymotic diseases. Of these 1 was from scarlet fever, 2 were from diphtheria. 9 from whooping cough, 4 from enteric fever, and 3 from diarrhœa. These deaths give a zymotic rate of 0·7 per 1,000.

The deaths of infants under one year of age amounted to 67, or about 22 per cent. of the total number at all ages, and measured by their ratio to the births registered during the quarter, were in the proportion of 104 per 1,000.

The following is the return of infectious diseases notified during the quarter: Small-pox 0, scarlet fever 45, diphtheria 5, enteric fever 5, puerperal fever 1 ; total 56.

C. W. PHILPOT, M.D., LOND.,
Medical Officer of health

Vol. VI. No. 51.

The death rate declined in the first 30 years of the nineteenth century but, as the following figures show, in certain places increased again between 1831 and 1841. These figures are taken from Chadwick's report.

	1831	1841
	(per 1000 people)	
Birmingham	14.6	27.2
Leeds	20.7	27.2
Bristol	16.9	31.0
Manchester	30.2	33.0
Liverpool	21	34.8

Which town's death rate has increased the most? Why does Manchester show the smallest increase (see The Industrial Town for clues). Remember that these figures give the average; in the most densely populated parts of the town the death rate would have been much higher.

UNNECESSARY DEATH

In the 1842 report Chadwick sought to shock his readers:

> The deaths caused during one year in England and Wales by epidemic, endemic and contagious disease, including fever, typhus and scarletina, amounting to 56,461, the greatest proportion of which are proved to be preventible, it may be said that the effect is as if the whole county of Westmoreland or Huntingdonshire . . . were either depopulated annually.

Look back in the book and see how Chadwick believed that deaths from preventible diseases could be avoided.

	Measles.	Pyaemia.	Scarlet Fever.	Typhoid Fever.	Diarrhoea.	Erysipelas.	Diphtheria.	Whooping Cough.	Total.
All Saints	...	...	...	...	...	...	...	1	1
St. Michael's	...	...	...	1	...	...	1	...	2
St. Aldate's	...	...	...	...	2	...	...	1	3
St. Ebbe's	1	...	...	3	2	...	...	5	11
St. Thomas'	2	...	...	2	5	...	...	...	9
Jericho	1	...	...	2	2	...	...	2	7
Magdalen	...	1	...	...	2	2	...	4	9
Cowley St. John	4	...	...	1	2	1	...	10	18
St. Clement's	1	...	1	...	1	...	...	6	9
St. Giles'	1	1	...	2	...	1	...	1	6
Osney	1	...	1	4	2	...	1	1	10
Hincksey	...	...	1	...	1	...	...	2	4
St. Peter-le-Bailey	...	...	...	...	2	...	...	1	3
New Botley	...	...	...	...	...	1	...	...	1
	11	2	3	15	21	5	2	34	93

The M.O.H. Report of deaths from infectious diseases in Oxford for 1884. Which was the most serious infectious disease?

PRESTON IN 1844

The Rev. John Clay reported on Preston in the first report of the Inquiry into the State of Large Towns and Populous Districts in 1844:

> . . . the mortality of the town chiefly predominates among the children of the working classes, the mortality among them increased as the social condition of the parent sinks . . . additional causes are connected with the ignorance, indifference, neglect, or selfishness of the parents. Their ignorance leads them to give their offspring the most improper food even when they are able to procure for them wholesome sustenance; and too often the child is destroyed by the gin poured into it with the intent to "nourish it".

How could the problem he outlined be solved?

The 1848 Public Health Act

The opponents of the Bill were either those who felt that there would be unnecessary expense on the rates or those who feared the loss of local control to Westminster. A letter to the *Morning Chronicle* on 20 April 1848 expressed the fear:

> Editor
>   Even in Constantinople or Grand Cairo where plague and cholera are decimating the population it is doubtful whether such a bill would be desirable.
>   A Ratepayer

Opposition was also expressed in Lincoln in the same year. This extract comes from S.E. Finer's *Life and Times of Sir Edwin Chadwick* (1952):

In 1847 Lord Morpeth introduced a Public Health Bill in Parliament, which stated that "further and more effectual provision ought to be made for improving the sanitary condition of towns and populous places in England and Wales". Local boards were to be set up to look after public health.

> Landlords of houses, men who have raised themselves by trade to some degree of independence and have built a lot of cottages . . . they are retired tradesmen generally . . . they are afraid of expenses which as landlords they would be called upon to pay.

Bromley Town Hall. After its opening in 1865 the Bromley local board moved into part of it. It was dubbed "the Board's Palace".

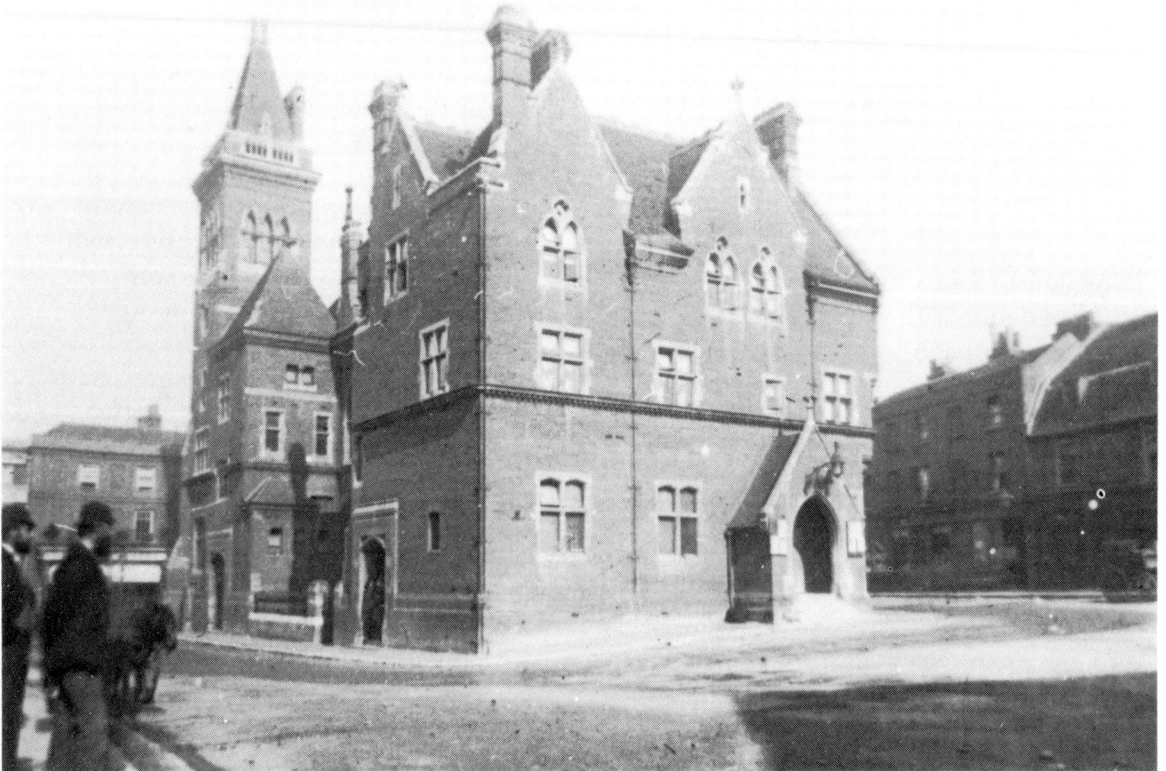

HOW THE BOARDS WERE FORMED

The Bill was defeated, but the following year a second, weaker one was passed. As a result of the opposition the Act did not make the setting up of local boards compulsory. A local board could be formed when the death rate reached 23 per thousand of population. However, Chadwick feared opposition to the formation of a local board, or where a local petition was drawn up, and he expressed this fear in a letter to Lord Morpeth on 21 July 1848:

> I know places in the North where two or three manufacturers may, by their influence with the ratepayers, almost effectively prevent any application whatsoever. Then all the butchers, all the fishmongers, all the poulterers who are to be subjected to inspection, all the lodging-house keepers, all the owners of the classes of houses having cellar tenements, and persons carrying on trades which are nuisances, must be in

> array against the Bill – all these are ratepayers: and the others of the middle classes who will be frightened with stories and the increase in rates.

Why did he feel that these groups might oppose a local board?

THE BROMLEY LOCAL BOARD

By 1854 only 182 local boards of health had been set up. But gradually, as fever or even cholera outbreaks led to a sharp increase in the death rate, more local parishes set up boards.

The population of Bromley in Kent had been rapidly increasing, and the new residents improved trade. After the cholera outbreak of 1865-6, however, the death rate rose alarmingly and it was feared that this would affect trade. Dr William Farr, the Medical Adviser of the Vestry, said in 1867:

> To defer would not save expense. The result would be houses run-up without inspection, cholera would come and then in the excitement of the moment, something would be done.

Arguments such as this won the day, and in the same year a local board was formed.

Many of Chadwick's fears for the loss of local control to central government were justified. Under the Act a General Board of Health had been established for five years to supervise newly formed local boards. Unfortunately it was not continued because people feared control from London.

Try and find out if there was a local board in your area. The local newspapers of the time will be useful.

CESS-CUM-POOLTON

Charles Dickens writing in *Household Words* in 1853 mocked the opposition:

> Ratepayers of Cess-cum-Poolton! Rally round your vested interests. Health is enormously expensive. Introduce the Public Health Act and you will be pauperized! Be filthy and be fat, cess-pools and constitutional government! Gases and Glory! No insipid water!!! . . . Reason with you? No, we won't do that, we are not talking about reason but about rates . . .

Local Health Officials

The latter part of the century saw the appointment of full-time officials, known as medical officers of health (M.O.H.), to supervise health problems in their areas. Their appointment was compulsory and the powers which they held were sometimes resented.

CHADWICK'S RECOMMENDATIONS

The bulk of the investigations for the 1842 *Report on Sanitary Conditions of the Labouring Population* were carried out by Poor Law doctors. In his conclusion Chadwick recommended

> . . . that for the prevention of the disease occasioned by defective ventilation, and other causes by impuring in places of work and other places where large numbers are assembled, and for the general promotion of the means necessary to prevent disease, that it would be good economy to appoint a district medical officer, independent of private practice, and with the securities of special qualifications and responsibilities to initiate sanitary measures . . .

Why did Chadwick believe that a well-qualified, full-time medical officer of health (M.O.H.) would "be good economy" [save money]?

THE DUTIES OF THE MEDICAL OFFICER

Liverpool was the first town to appoint an M.O.H., Dr Duncan, in 1847. In the following year the Public Health Act allowed local boards to appoint M.O.H.s. They were made compulsory in London in 1855, but not in the rest of the country until 1872. The M.O.H. for London, Sir John Simon, drew up a list of duties. These were published in *The Times* on 24 December 1855:

THE INSPECTOR OF NUISANCES

The Lambeth M.O.H.'s report of 1888 described the improvements which had taken place in the quality of inspectors since 1855.

> The Inspector was [in 1855] an unskilled workman holding that which might almost be regarded as a sinecure office, an official recruited into the service of the vestry from the ranks of ex-sailors, ex-policemen, or army pensioners . . . . A knowledge of sanitary matters acquired from a course of technical training was not expected of him.

By 1888 better qualifications were needed and the job had expanded:

> . . . the Inspector of today is a man highly trained and skilled in plumbing,

> The Officer of Health is appointed in order that through him the local sanitary authority may be duly informed of such influences as are setting against the healthiness of his district, and of such steps as medical science can advise for their removal; secondly, to execute such special functions as may devolve upon him . . . and thirdly, to contribute to the general stock of knowledge with regard to the sanitary condition of the people.

The M.O.H. was invaluable to the town council because he was able to present expert advice. But his powers were sometimes resented. Which groups might the M.O.H. offend if he was too keen in his duties?

Nuisances dealt with in Oxford. Which nuisances ▷ were the most common, and which the most serious?

drain laying, and the allied handicrafts and other technical duties of his profession.

Why do you think that better qualified officials contributed to a fall in the London death rate?

DUTIES OF THE INSPECTOR OF NUISANCES

The Lambeth Medical Officer's Report of 1888 looked at the duties involved:

a. **regular day to day duties, having a temporary effect**
   – inspection of bakehouses, schools and lodging houses, the investigation of nuisance complaints . . . paperwork, attendance at court.

b. **supervision of work leading to permanent improvement**
   – supervision of drainage improvement work, paving, and draining of yards, supervision and improvement of water supply and sanitary equipment.

The M.O.H. commented that in the 1850s the inspector regarded his work completed when the nuisance had been removed. By 1888 his task was not ended until the whole dwelling had been put into a satisfactory and healthy condition.

Another table from the Sheffield M.O.H.'s Report of ▷ 1877. Look at the Sheffield O.S. extract on page 8 and the table on page 25. Why did so many houses not have either back doors or rear windows?

Which departments and officials are responsible for public health in your area today? What powers do they have?

DESCRIPTION OF NUISANCES ABATED AND THE NUMBER OF HOUSES AFFECTED THEREBY.

Description of Nuisances.	After Notice from Committee.	After Notice from Inspector.	Total.
Privy vaults emptied and filled in, and w.c's. constructed, and the drains connected with the sewer	21	4	25
Privy vaults emptied only in district without drainage	..	14	14
Water laid on to, and defective water supply to closets remedied	55	20	75
Blocked and defective closets repaired	36	22	58
Scullery drains disconnected by syphon trap	34	9	43
Blocked and defective drains repaired, i.e., new traps, &c.	67	20	87
Water laid on to houses (or pumps repaired)	20		20
Dirty and dilapidated premises cleansed & repaired	61		61
House drains connected with sewer not previously connected	11		11
Offensive accumulations removed	15	40	55
Animals kept so as to be a nuisance removed	35		35
Defective urinals repaired	2	4	6
Overcrowded premises relieved	3		3
Closet accommodation provided	1		1
Closets improperly placed removed	9		9
Number of persons summoned before Justices			4
Number of rooms fumigated after infectious diseases			70
Articles disinfected from rooms, including beds, mattresses, pillows, blankets, carpets, &c.			371
Privies and house drains, &c., removed from polluting river, under Rivers Pollution Act.	9		9

THOS. J. HULL,
Inspector of Nuisances.

March 30th, 1885.

CONSTRUCTION AND VENTILATION OF HOUSES.

No. of Group.	Ventilation of Houses.				Percentage of Houses.			
	Without Backdoors.	Without Back Windows.	With Sash Windows Opening.	With Casement Windows.	Without Backdoors.	Without Back Windows.	With Sash Windows Opening.	With Casement Windows.
1	220	202	64	151	60·3	55·6	17·6	41·5
2	313	274	62	66	78·6	68·8	15·5	16·5
3	673	637	226	246	70·7	67·5	18·2	19·8
4	411	393	90	101	77·4	74·0	16·9	19·0
5	365	353	48	164	68·7	66·5	9·0	30·9
6	340	317	28	150	68·6	64·0	5·6	30·3
7	382	389	3	137	89·4	90·8	0·7	32·0
8	178	149	53	97	64·2	53·7	19·1	31·4
9	149	140	43	160	33·4	31·3	9·6	35·8
10	284	275	4	94	71·7	69·4	1·0	23·
11	201	·200	35	32	68·3	68·0	11·9	10·5
Totals	3716	3528	656	1398	*68·9	*65·4	*12·2	*25·9

* NOTE.—Percentages in the entire Area.

Hospitals

Charles Knight in the *Cyclopaedia of London*, published in 1851, described the people who sought treatment in city hospitals:

> The majority of persons received as patients into the London hospitals are mechanics, labourers, reduced tradesmen, or servants. There are, however, admissions of individuals of both sexes, and particularly, of the very lowest class of society and of the worst character: this is unavoidable, and care is taken to repress and as far as possible to punish improper conduct . . . . In all ordinary cases it is necessary that an applicant for admission should obtain the recommendation of a governor [i.e. an official or subscriber] by his signature to a printed petition, of which forms are to be procured at the hospital. Many are admitted without any other recommendation than the urgency of their case. Cases of accident are admitted on all days, at any hour whatever.

Which groups does this hospital cater for?

After 1834 each Poor Law union that was formed had its own hospital, attached to the workhouse, where inmates and those on out-relief were taken when seriously ill. Other hospitals were maintained by various charities and by public subscription. The comfortably off were able to attend private hospitals where they paid the full cost.

A WORKHOUSE HOSPITAL

The workhouse infirmary (hospital) was often the only place for the poor. A missionary describes his work in the St Pancras infirmary:

> In the infirmary wards the work is equally hard, and our experience is, that the strongest men break down after a few years and have to be removed . . . as it is from bed to bed work, and as many of the sufferers are deaf, loud reading and speaking is required all day long. Our visitor in the Holborn Union writes "During the year there have been 437 deaths in the House. With all these I had read individually." (Quoted in *These Fifty Years*, 1884, by J.M. Weylland)

Why were most of the patients deaf?

A HOSPITAL VISITOR

Between 1846 and 1864 Mr Kaines worked for the London City Mission. He described his experiences as a visitor at the Islington Fever Hospital in 1847.

> There has been a larger proportion than usual of cases of scarlet fever, inducing putridity [infection]. I have had the peculiar feeling on my palate for days together, and have been obliged to take medicine to get rid of it.

> Several of our nurses have died during the year, and as many as three medical men were brought down with fever at one time; one of them is slowly recovering from a third attack. Is it not a mercy and a blessing that I should have been spared? (*These Fifty Years*)

The hospital had 250 beds. In one year 556 patients died. Why would Mr Kaines be so welcome in the hospital?

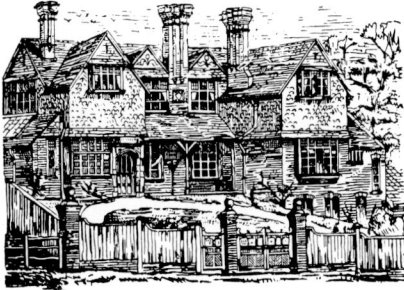

NORWOOD COTTAGE HOSPITAL,
Hermitage Road, Central Hill.

PRESIDENTS—
James Watney, Esq., M.P.,   William Grantham, Esq., Q.C., M.P.

COMMITTEE OF MANAGEMENT—
Rev. R. Allen, Captain J. B. Clay, E. Colegrave, Esq., J. Judd, Esq., F.R. Hist. S.
A. McAnally, Esq., G. W. Paine, Esq., H. Sutherland, Esq.,
S. Symons, Esq.,   Rev. James Watson.

Hon. Treasurer—General R. Ranken.   Hon. Solicitor—G. H. Finch, Esq.

Hon. Auditors—Wm. Smith, Esq.,   W. H. Steere, Esq.

Bankers—The London and South Western Bank, Limited, Westow Hill,
Upper Norwood, S.E.

Hon. Secretaries—
Frederick Clift, Esq., LL.D., Sylcot, Norwood, S.E.
Henry Phillips, Esq., 1, Gatestone, Road, Norwood, S.E.

The Hospital is intended for the benefit of persons engaged in industrial occupations (including domestic servants) who are unable to obtain medical attention, accommodation, and nursing at their own homes, and for accidents of all kinds and cases of sudden illness (non-infectious). The benefits of the Institution are extended to Norwood and the surrounding district. The admission of patients—except when provisionally admitted, shall be by Letters of Recommendation. The Hospital is supported by Annual Subscriptions, Donations, Bequests, payments made by Patients, &c. Every Donor, past or future, of ten

NORWOOD
COTTAGE HOSPITAL,
HERMITAGE ROAD,
CENTRAL HILL.

PRESIDENTS :
JAMES WATNEY, Jun., Esq., M.P.
WILLIAM GRANTHAM, Esq., Q.C., M.P.

MEDICAL STAFF :
J. BROCKWELL, Esq.   HENRY HETLEY, Esq.
J. GALTON, Esq.   R. M. MILLER, Esq.
WM. GANDY, Esq.   J. SHARMAN, Esq.

HON. TREASURER :
GENERAL R. RANKEN.

HON. SECRETARIES :
FREDERICK CLIFT, Esq., LL.D., Syclot, Norwood, S.E.
HENRY PHILLIPS, Esq., 1, Gatestone Road, Norwood, S.E.

————:0:————

Founded in 1882, for the relief of the Sick Poor of the District.

Donations and Subscriptions, which are earnestly solicited, may be paid to the LONDON AND SOUTH WESTERN BANK, Limited, Westow Hill, Norwood, S.E., or to the Hon. Treasurer, General R. RANKEN, Eskmount, Highfield Hill, Norwood, S.E.

The Report, containing full details of the working of the Hospital during the past year, may be obtained on application to any of the Officers.

THE WHITECHAPEL HOSPITAL

Montague Williams in *Round London*, published in 1894, described this hospital in the Whitechapel Road in the East End of London:

The hospital consists of a large building facing the Whitechapel Road, from which it is divided by a courtyard, which serves as a carriage-way. The main entrance leads into the receiving room, which . . . was opened last June.

. . . There is a matron, and there are nearly 30 sisters, and over 200 nurses. Some 10 physicians, and an equal number of surgeons, are aided by a large staff of junior surgeons and dressers.

Four separate rooms constitute a ward, and each room contains about 52 or 56 beds, on an emergency 76 beds can be made up. As a rule between 600 –

These two extracts from Burdett's Directory of Upper Norwood, Penge and Anerley *for 1886 illustrate the type of information you can get from local directories. Which groups did the hospital cater for?*

700 are occupied. On each floor there are some 13 or 15 nurses and one sister. Communications between the doctors and nurses on the one hand, and the patients on the other, have very largely to be conducted by signs and symbols.

Communication between hospital staff and patients was difficult here because many of the patients were European Jews, recently arrived in Britain from Germany, Russia, etc.

Try and identify the hospitals in your area. How many of them are Victorian? The local directories will be useful for detail and advertisements.

The Peabody Buildings

We have seen the problems faced by the poor in finding rooms to rent which were not a danger to their health in the growing cities and towns. The earliest improvements came from various charities which built large dwelling blocks. Later, town councils began to build what we now call council houses or flats.

PEABODY BUILDINGS

It was to meet these needs that George Peabody, a wealthy American banker, first gave money for housing in 1862. A trust was formed and, today, Peabody Buildings can still be seen in London. *The Times*, on 11 January 1866, described the Shadwell Estate:

> Drainage and ventilation have been insured with the utmost possible care; the instant removal of dust is effected by means of shafts which descend from every corridor to cellars in the basement, whence it is carted away; the passages are all kept clean and lighted with gas . . . water from cisterns is distributed by pipes into every tenement and there are baths free for all who desire to use them. Laundries, with wringing machines and drying lofts, are at the service of every inmate . . . . Every living room or kitchen is abundantly provided with cupboards, shelving, and other conveniences, and each fireplace includes a boiler and oven. But what gratifies the tenant [most] . . . are the ample and airy spaces which serve as playgrounds for their children . . . under their mothers' eye, and safe from the risk of passing carriages and laden carts.

List the ways in which these buildings are much healthier than the slums.

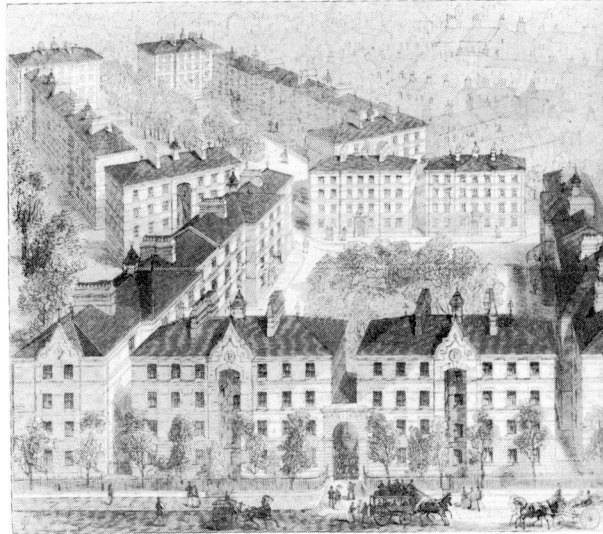

Peabody Square, Blackfriars Road, London, opened in 1871. These were more spacious than his earlier flats and had no corridors. (Illustrated London News, *1872*)

THE TENANTS

In the *Annual Report of the Peabody Trust* for 1865 the occupations of the tenants were listed as

> Charwomen, monthly nurses, basket-makers, butchers, carpenters, firemen, labourers, porters, omnibus drivers, sempstresses, shoe-makers, tailors, waiters, warehousemen, watch finishers, turners, staymakers, smiths, sawyers, printers, painters, laundresses, letter carriers, artificial flower-makers, dressmakers, carmen, cabinet-makers, book-binders, and others.

Look up the occupations that you do not recognize. At the time there was criticism that the Trust was not catering for the really poor, defined by Charles Booth as those who earned less than 21s. a week. The majority of the Peabody tenants earned between 20s. and 30s. a week and paid 4s.9d. in rent.

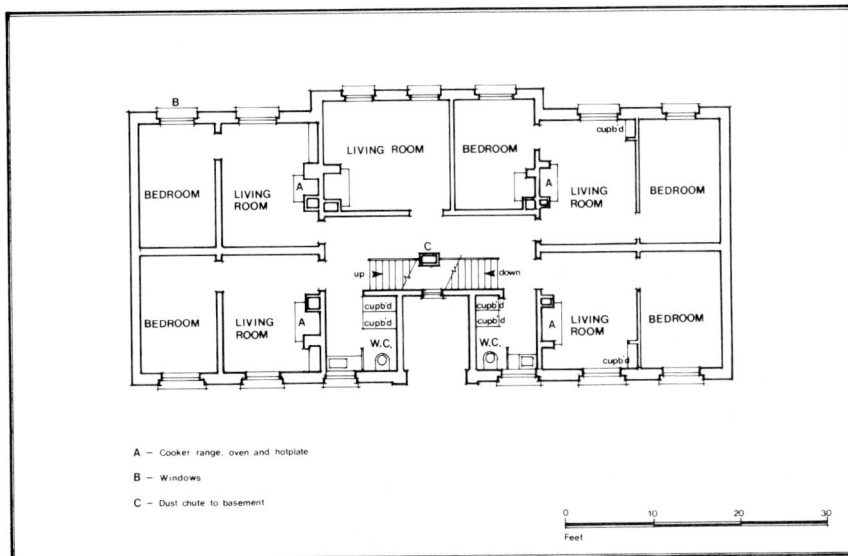

A — Cooker range, oven and hotplate

B — Windows

C — Dust chute to basement

0   10   20   30
Feet

A plan of a floor in one of the Peabody Square buildings. The bathroom was situated on the ground floor and the W.C. was shared. How many families did each identical floor contain and how many rooms did each family have? (Clue: only the main doors are shown.)

THE TRUST'S REGULATIONS

These included:

1. No applicants for rooms will be entertained unless every member of the applicant's family has been vaccinated . . .
2. The rents will be paid weekly in advance.
3. No arrears will be allowed.
4. The passages, steps, closets, and lavatory windows must be washed every Saturday and swept every morning before 10 o'clock . . .
5. Washing must be done in the laundry only . . .
6. No carpets, mats, etc., will be permitted to be beaten or shaken after 10 o'clock in the morning. Refuse must not be thrown out of doors or windows.
7. Tenants must pay all costs of repairs and of damage in their rooms.
8. Children will not be allowed to play on the stairs, in the passages, or in the laundries.
9. Dogs must not be kept on the premises.
10. Tenants cannot be allowed to paper, paint, or drive nails into the walls. ·
11. No tenant will be allowed to under-let or take in lodgers.
12. Disorderly and intemperate tenants will receive immediate notice to quit.
13. The gas will be turned off at 11 p.m. and the outer doors closed for the night [tenants had keys].
14. Tenants are required to report to the superintendent any births, deaths, or infectious diseases occurring in their rooms . . .

The rules were felt to be severe. Which of the rules would seem strange to the majority of new tenants? How do they reflect the growing ideas for public health?

The Water Supply

Chadwick had shown in the 1840s the need for a constant supply of pure water to each house but, as we have seen, supplying water to the poor was not always profitable to the various private water companies. By the end of the century conditions had improved. In 1889 only just over half the houses in London were supplied with water. By 1900 this had been improved to 95 per cent.

THE INCENTIVES TO CHANGE

The M.O.H. for Wandsworth in 1866 commented on the recent cholera epidemic.

> In the treatment of the latter epidemic, it became manifest to everyone concerned, that no measure was more needed than the supply of this necessity of life upon what is called the constant service principle; and it is still further believed that no other system of supply is calculated in so great a degree to arrest the progress of any future epidemic, and to preserve the health of the people at large.

Why was a constant supply of water so important to health?

ARGUMENT OVER EDINBURGH'S WATER SUPPLIES

In the 1860s pressure began for the city to take over the major water company because of the poor supply.

The company's defence

The following letter was written by the manager of the water company to the town council:

> Dear Sir,
> ... Now if you will enquire carefully where complaints come from you will find it exclusively from tenements where interruption has arisen from a temporary cause .... Unfortunately, however, in the whole, or nearly the whole, of the vast number of houses built, for occupancy in separate flats, the supply of water is furnished by a ½″ or ¾″ pipe, for the use of the whole of the occupants, consisting seldom of less than eight, and frequently as many as 20, 30 or 40 separate families.
> I am etc.
>
> Alex. Ramsey

I have omitted the final paragraph. Can you guess what it said (clue: pipe and numbers)?

The company is to blame!

David Lewis in *Edinburgh's Water Supply* (1908) described his work as a reforming councillor some 40 years before:

> [I] had at first believed there was some force in it [the company's argument]. Careful investigation, however, had led to my changing this opinion entirely. An examination of the cisterns in such houses as referred to proved the contrary .... In one of these the cistern was quite dry, with cobwebs on the bottom of it .... A practical plumber called in ... declared the apparatus perfect and complete.

Before you make a final decision on whether the water company was to blame for the poor supply of water, read the following letter of the 24 June 1869 from a resident in Chessel's Court complaining of the shortage of water over the past five years.

I reside close to the brewery, and I have plenty of water on the Sunday when the brewery is not operating.

Heated meetings

In 1871 various meetings took place concerning the council's proposals to use St Mary's Loch to increase the supply of water. At one meeting on the 17 June 1871 John McVey, a plasterer, spoke for the scheme:

Was it those who were working for a weekly wage, and who laboured from early morning till late at night, he asked, and who were crying out about the silence? No! it was those who lived in luxury and ease ...

Another meeting, this time against the Bill, was held on the same day.

Working-men of Edinburgh, Leith and Portobello, your presence is earnestly invited to give expression to your condemnation of this unnecessary water scheme, and of the policy of those "Liberal Representatives" who are spending your money in thousands in violation of every principle of representative government, and in defiance of the declared will of the constituents.

What arguments were being put forward? Which might you have sympathized with if you had been a working man?

This particular scheme was defeated, but a compromise was eventually put forward and agreed.

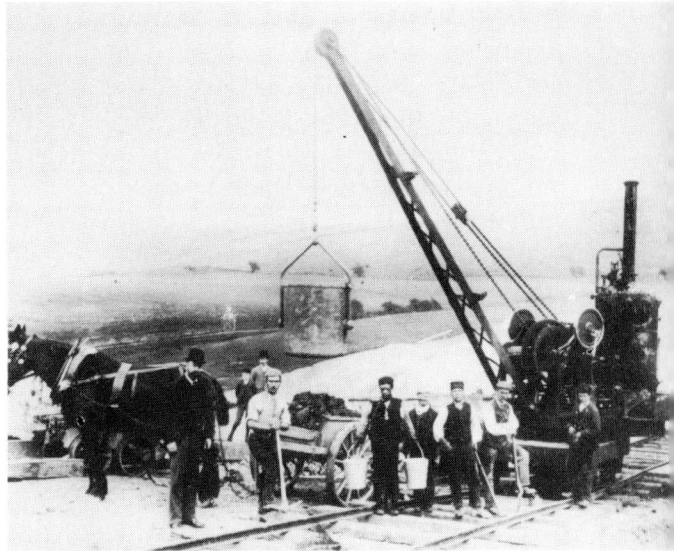

The building of Clough Boltan Reservoir, East Lancashire in 1895. In what ways did reservoir construction alter the landscape?

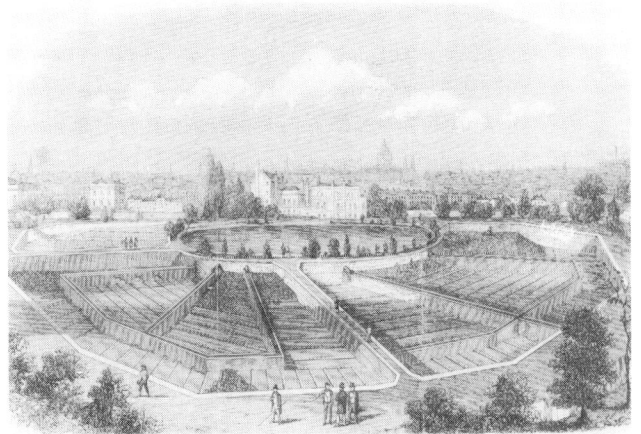

The New River Water Works, London, 1856. The water overflows from the central reservoir into the beds through a filtering layer of sand. This was one of the early attempts to provide safe water for London. (Illustrated London News, 1856)

Try and find out how your town is supplied with water. Is there still a local water works or reservoir?

Redevelopment in Croydon

In the nineteenth century Croydon was a rapidly growing town, well served by railways to London. Its mediaeval market area, known as Middle Row, had been built over and by mid-century was an area of small streets and houses in a very poor state of repair.

A NIGHT IN MIDDLE ROW

On 30 June 1881 a reporter for the *Croydon Advertiser* spent from 11.30 a.m. Saturday until Sunday night in Middle Row. He was very critical of reporters from other Croydon papers who conducted short interviews with the inhabitants, often holding handkerchiefs soaked in camphor or ___

A LODGING HOUSE IN THE OLD TOWN, 1861

The 1861 census showed that roughly half the houses in this area had become lodging houses and beer houses. A typical one housed the following people:

Name	Relation to Head of Household	Condition	Age	Occupation	Place of birth
Charles Stagg	Head	M(arried)	29	Beer house keeper	Croydon
Mary Stagg	Wife	"	37		Cliffe, Kent
Charles Stagg	Son		3		Croydon
Baby	Son		2 days		Croydon
Emma Bailey	Niece		15	General servant	Dudley, Staffs
Elizabeth Bailey	Nurse	Widow	66	Monthly nurse	Rochester, Kent
Duncan Page	Lodger	M	64	Gardener	Scotland
James Wilton	"	"	52	Painter	Godalming, Surrey
James Sevena	"	"	33	Brushmaker	Maidstone, Kent
Ann Sevena	"	Wife	36		Woolwich, Kent
George Burton	"	U(married)	43	Umbrella maker	Surrey
Thomas Shingleton	"	W(idower)	48	Labourer	Seaford, Sussex
John Green	Lodger	U	28	Artisan	Ipswich, Suffolk
Michael Miller	"	M	28	Labourer	Bletchingley, Surrey
James Edwards	"	M	56	Carpenter	Caterham, Surrey
Thomas Ede	"	U	39	Stone mason	Reigate, Surrey

How many people are living in the house? What sort of occupations do they follow? What is interesting about their place of birth?

The Middle Row area development plan of 1889. This sketch is taken from the original. The shaded area was demolished and the black line indicates the new street patterns. What advantages did the redevelopment bring?

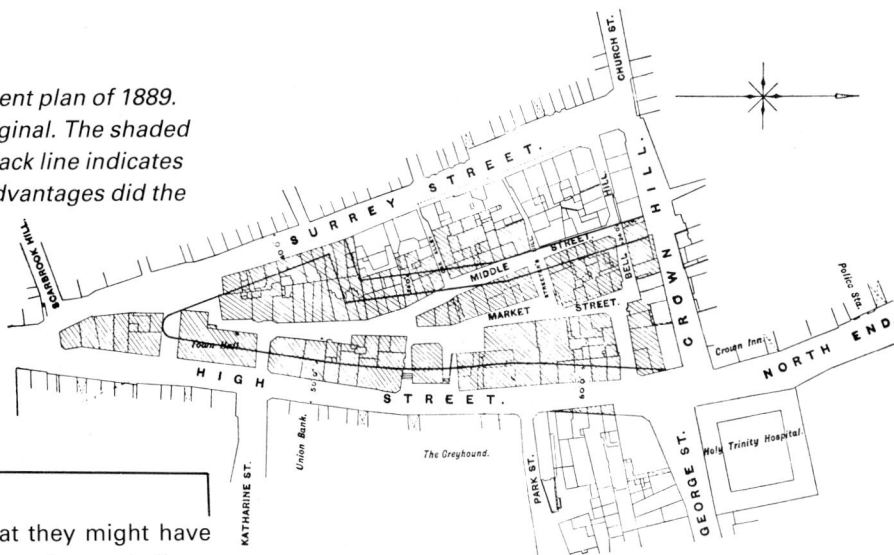

eau de cologne. He thought that they might have just as well written about the area from a balloon directly above! In his conclusion he wrote:

> . . . the greatest danger was the commoness itself; here people are herded together . . . . The air of the room must be germ laden and dangerous . . . and the stench permeating the immediate vicinity is too well known to need description.

CONDEMNATION OF MIDDLE ROW

In 1884 a council committee was formed to consider the widening of the High Street and the destruction of the worst of Middle Row (see plan). *The Croydon Advertiser* supported the proposed improvement and on 2 June 1888 recorded:

> Within thirty feet of the principal hotel in the borough there exists a human moral piggery that, for low depravity, either Newcastle or Manchester might match, but certainly could not surpass . . . . One gentleman, residing himself in a charming house on the banks of the Thames, is the happy owner of no lesss than 14 residences in Middle Row . . .

Why did the newspaper not reveal the absentee landlord's name?

RIVAL ARGUMENTS

On 30 June 1888 the *Croydon Guardian* objected to the demolition of Middle Row:

> . . . on precisely the same grounds on which we opposed the establishment of Free Libraries, the utter injustice in forcing the payment of these things on those who do not ask for them and do participate in them.

On the same day the *Croydon Advertiser* wrote:

> The important subject of widening the narrow part of the High Street, Croydon and abolishing that den of infamy, known as Middle-Row, came before the Croydon Town Council at its meeting last Monday evening at the Town Hall.

Which paper was in favour of the improvement and which against? How do you know?

The photograph on page 10 shows Middle Row *c.* 1890. In that year an Improvement Act was gained giving the council the right to purchase land in the triangle marked on the plan. Demolition began in 1893. This section illustrates the way in which you can use local newspapers.

41

Improvements by 1900

Improvements did not come by chance, but as a result of hard work on the part of many reformers. Certainly by the end of the century many changes had occurred.

THE PUBLIC INTEREST

One man, Sir John Simon, deserves a place along with Chadwick in the history of public health. Simon was the M.O.H. for London and he believed that poverty was among the worst of sanitary evils. He also believed that property rights often stood in the way of reform. In *English Sanitary Institutions* (1890) he wrote:

> The factory chimney that eclipses the light – the melting house that nauseates an entire parish, the slaughterhouse that forms round itself a dangerous circle of diseases – these surely are not private, but public affairs . . . and as for the rights of property – they are pecuniary [financial]. Life too is a great property.

How do you think this view would have been received by businessmen and manufacturers?

HOPES FOR THE FUTURE

In the *History of the Great Peace* (1858) Harriet Martineau wrote:

> The attention given to sanitary improvement is a leading feature of our time. Thirty years ago, scarcely anybody thought of pure air, good drainage, a sufficient supply of water, or even cleanliness of person, as we all think of them now.

She concluded:

> Before the history of another period shall be written by some one of the next generation, we may hope that the Thames will have ceased to receive the filth of London and of other towns; that the sewers will answer their proper purpose; that every house will be supplied with pure water; that the dead will be buried in country cemeteries; that every stagnant ditch and dunghill will be treated as a public offence; and that the causes of fever will be destroyed wherever it is possible to detect them.

Which of her hopes would you have considered the most important if you had been living then? From the information given in previous sections, see how many of her hopes were to be realized by 1900.

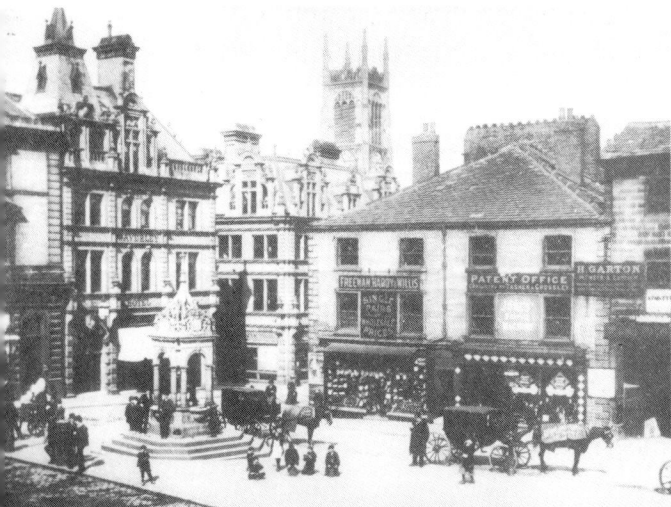

Leeds in the late nineteenth century. Can you pick out the new buildings from the old? How can you tell? What did the fountain erected in 1887 commemorate?

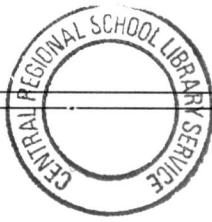

IMPROVEMENTS IN BIRMINGHAM

Birmingham in the 1870s was one of the most progressive cities. Under its mayor, Joseph Chamberlain, it reduced its death rate considerably by improving water supplies and encouraging slum clearance.

In 1881 the Town Council could report:

> Birmingham is now, as regards its health, first among all the large towns of Great Britain which are comparable to it . . .

In 1875 the Artisan's Dwelling Act was passed which enabled councils compulsorily to purchase land for redevelopment. Birmingham was one of the first to do this. Some argued that insufficient working class housing was being built on the sites of the cleared slums but Arthur Hickmott in *Houses for the People* (1897) showed that they were providing some:

> Ryder Street – In order to replace the people displaced by the improvement scheme of some years earlier, the Council in the years 1890 to 1892 erected 103 dwellings of the cottage type, accommodating about 500 persons, let at 5s. to 6s. 3d. per week. They are five-roomed dwellings, substantially built, and cost about £175 each. The buildings have back doors opening on an enclosed brick-paved yard, 36 feet across. The houses at 5s. 6d. have on the ground floor, a living room 13 feet square, and a kitchen 12 feet by 9 feet, fitted with an iron sink and a small copper [boiler]. There is also a pantry and a coal cupboard. On the first floor there are two bedrooms, and above them, a spacious well-lighted attic. Good grates and ovens are provided in every house, and iron is used for mantelpieces and other fittings. Each house has a penny-in-the slot gas meter, and a flushed W.C. . . .

List the improvements which these two-bedroomed terraced houses contain compared with the back to backs of the earlier years.

Imagine you were a poor child living in a major industrial town in 1900. In what ways would life have been more comfortable for you then than if you had been born at the beginning of the nineteenth century?

An advertisement from Holts's Guide to Sutton, Surrey *of 1896. How does it reflect the developments which had taken place?*

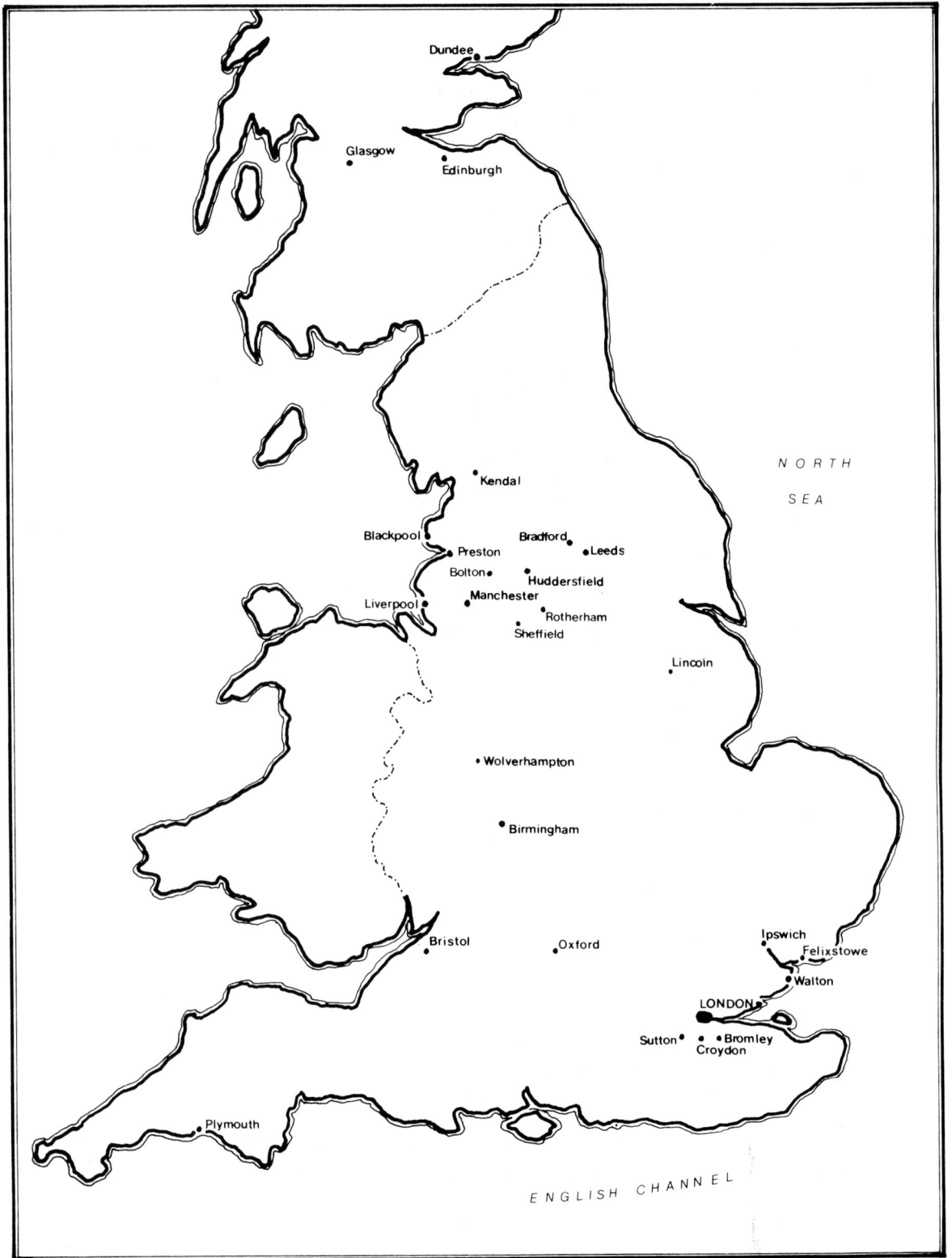

NORTH
SEA

Dundee

Glasgow
Edinburgh

Kendal

Blackpool
Bradford
Preston
Leeds
Bolton
Huddersfield
Liverpool
Manchester
Rotherham
Sheffield

Lincoln

Wolverhampton

Birmingham

Bristol
Oxford
Ipswich
Felixstowe
Walton
LONDON
Sutton
Bromley
Croydon

Plymouth

ENGLISH CHANNEL

Difficult Words

artisan	a mechanic, usually a town worker.
bacillus	a disease-causing bacteria.
back-to-back housing	rows of terraced houses built back to back to save space. Thus on three sides there were no windows and hence no ventilation.
bone and bottle shops	shops for the poor.
cesspool	a pool or pit used where the house does not have main drainage.
cholera	highly infectious and deadly disease.
cistern	a tank for holding water.
contagious	a disease spread by direct contact.
dunghill	a heap of dung (manure, excreta).
dyehouse	building in which dyeing is done.
dysentery	a contagious disease; the symptoms are vomiting and diarrhorea.
endemic	prevalent or regularly found in a particular area or amongst a certain group.
enteric fever	infectious fever caused by a bacillus characterized by fever, rose red rash.
epidemic	a disease that attacks great numbers in one place at one time and often spreads.
farrier	one who shoes horses.
garret	an attic room; one just under the roof.
guano	the dung of sea-fowl, used as manure. Before artificial fertilizers it was imported from South America.
local board	an elected group who supervised health matters and could raise rates and introduce bye laws.
log book	daily diary kept by the headmaster.
M.O.H.	Medical Officer of Health.
miasma	foul smell (the miasmic theory was that disease was caused by smell).
midden	a dunghill or refuse tip.
National school	a school run by the Church of England.
night soil	the contents of privies or cesspools.
noxious	poisonous, harmful.
out relief	payment in money or kind given to the poor.
pestiferous	bringing the plague or disease.
Poor Law union	a group of parishes formed together after 1834 to supervise the poor in their area.
privy	a lavatory; may be no more than a hole in the ground in a shed draining into the cesspool.
Rookery	a slum.
sanitary	concerned with health.
scarlet fever	an infectious disease, marked by a sore throat and a red rash.
scavenger	a street cleaner.
sewage	refuse carried off by sewers.
sewerage	the system of sewers.
shippen	a cow-house or cattle shed, which was often attached to the house or cottage.
sinecure	a job without any work attached.
soup shop	where food, often soup, was given to the poor or unemployed.
speculative builder	one who takes a chance on his building, hoping for a quick profit.
tallow-chandler	a candle-maker.
tenement	strictly speaking, anything held; but usually a house or block divided between different families.

typhoid fever often confused with typhus because of the red spots.

typhus a dangerous fever transmitted by lice.

vestry a meeting of ratepayers elected to consider business in their parish.

zymotic an infectious disease.

Money

Always look at what money and wages could buy rather than at what seem low prices to us. It is no use butter being 4p a pound if we only earn 50p a week. Remember that there were 12 old pence (d.) in a shilling (s.) and 20 shillings to the pound. 6d. was the equivalent of 2½p, a shilling (1/-) 5p.

Date List

1831 Outbreak of cholera in Sunderland.

1832 13,000 died of cholera (one-third of whom were in London).

1834 The Poor Law Amendment Act. Doctors to be appointed to Poor Law unions.

1835 The Municipal Corporation Act, allowing for the establishment of local boards of health.

1838 Survey of the recent fever outbreak in Whitechapel.

1840 Smallpox vaccination provided free for children by the Poor Law guardians.

1842 *Report on The Sanitary Conditions of the Labouring Population* by Edwin Chadwick.

1844 No new back-to-back houses to be built in Manchester.

1844/5 Reports by the Health of Towns Commission.

1846 Nuisance Removals Act – but could only deal with existing nuisance *not* prevent it.

1847 First Medical Officer of Health appointed – Dr William Duncan, in Liverpool.

1848 Dr John Simon appointed M.O.H. for the City of London.

Public Health Act – General Board of Health formed.

Metropolitan Sewers Act.

1848/9 Cholera – 80,000 die (15,000 in London).

1852 Metropolitan Water Act – London's water not to be drawn from within five miles of the city.

1853 Compulsory vaccination for smallpox – but could not be enforced.

1855 Nuisance Removal Act – local boards could appoint Inspectors of Health.

1856 Metropolitan Board of Works for London.

1858 General Medical Council established – register to be kept.

1860 Moules' earth closet patented.

First Adulteration of Food Act (food not to have dangerous substances added).

1861 Regulations established for the training of nurses.

Prince Albert dies of cholera.

1863 Alkali Act – against water pollution, but limited effect.

1865/6 Third major cholera outbreak.

1868 Royal Sanitary Commission established (reported 1871).

Manchester appointed its first M.O.H.

Torren's Housing Act (Artisans' Dwelling Act) for the improvement or demolition of working-class dwellings and the building of new ones.

1870 First diploma in public health (from 1888 it was made compulsory for those officials in public health).
Smallpox epidemic – 44,000 die.
Further act for vaccination (becomes totally compulsory in 1898; in force till 1948).

1871 local government board established – to provide help and establish a central authority.

1872 M.O.H. compulsory.

1874 Registration Act – doctors required by law to sign certificates giving the cause of death.

1875 Compulsory notification of infectious diseases.
Public Health Act – brought together all previous legislation.
Artisans' Dwellings Act – whole areas could be redeveloped.
Sale of Food and Drugs Act.

1876 River Pollution Act – against water pollution.

1882 Robert Koch identifies the cholera baccillus.

1885 *Report of the Royal Commission for the Housing of the Working Classes*.

1890 Housing of the Working Classes Act – first effective legislation.

1892 Penny-in-the-slot gas meters invented.

1893 Cholera – 135 deaths.

1898 National Association for the Prevention of T.B. (tuberculosis) formed.

Bird, I., *Notes on Old Edinburgh*, 1869
Briggs, A., *Victorian Cities*, 1968
Chadwick, E., *Report on the Sanitary Conditions of the Labouring Population*, 1842
Chadwick, E., *Report on the System of Interments*, 1843
*Dickens, C., *Hard Times*, 1854
Dickens, C., *Household Words*, 1853
Diprose, J., *Some Accounts of the Parish of St. Clement Danes, London*, 1868
Engels, F., *Condition of the Working Class in England*, 1844
Finer, S.E., *Life and Times of Sir Edwin Chadwick*, 1952
*Gaskell, E., *North and South*, 1854
Henderson, W.O., *Industrial Britain under the Regency*, 1968
Knight, C., *Cyclopaedia of London*, 1851
Jobson, A., *Victorian Suffolk*, 1972
Lewis, D., *Edinburgh's Water Supply*, 1908
Longford, A.J., *A Centruy of Birmingham Life*, 1870
Mearns, W.C., *The Bitter Cry of Outcast London*, 1883
Palmer, R. (ed.), *A Touch of the Times*, 1974
Roberts, J., *Working Class Housing in Nineteenth Century Manchester*, c.1980
Roebuck, J., *Urban Development in Nineteenth Century London*, 1979
Simon, J., *English Sanitary Institutions*, 1890
Tarn, J.N., *Five Per Cent Philanthropy*, 1973
Wey11and, J.M., *These Fifty Years*, 1884
Williams, M., *Round London*, 1894
Williams, R., *London Rookeries and Colliers' Slums*, 1893
Wohl, A.S., *The Eternal Slum*, 1977

*Novels

=====Book List=====

There are very few books on this subject written specifically for children but two which are very useful are L. Rose, *Health and Hygiene*, Batsford, 1975, and R. Watson, *Edwin Chadwick. Poor Law and Public Health*, Longman, 1969.

The following volumes I found useful in writing this book.

Anon, *Pictorial History of Lancashire*, 1844
Anon, *Croydon: The story of a Hundred Years*, 1979
Besant, H., *London in the Nineteenth Century*, 1909